RESEARCH IN GENERAL PRACTICE

RESEARCH IN GENERAL PRACTICE

J.G.R. HOWIE

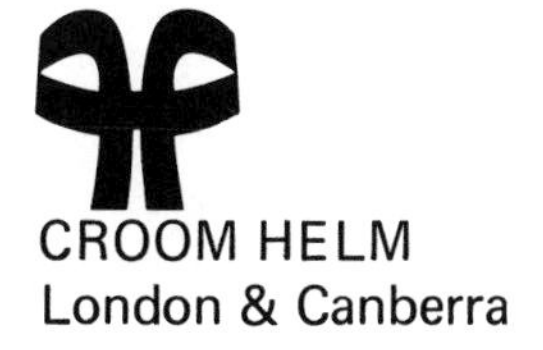

CROOM HELM
London & Canberra

Croom Helm Ltd, Provident House, Burrell Row,
Beckenham, Kent BR3 1AT
Croom Helm Australia Pty Ltd, 28 Kembla Street,
Fyshwick, ACT 2609, Australia
Reprinted 1983 and 1984

British Library Cataloguing in Publication Data

Howie, J.G.R.
Research in general practice.
1. Medical research – Great Britain
2. Physicians (General practice) –
Great Britain
I. Title
610'.72'041 R854.G7

ISBN 0-85664-506-0

Printed and bound in Great Britain by
Biddles Ltd, Guildford and King's Lynn

CONTENTS

ACKNOWLEDGEMENTS

This book represents the end point of several years spent thinking about and doing research. Many friends and colleagues – inside and outside general practice – have contributed generously to the ideas and projects described in the pages which follow and it is a pleasure to express my thanks to them here. None have helped more than my colleagues in the Aberdeen Department of General Practice and my indebtedness is greatest to Ian Richardson who, in addition, has kindly written the foreword, John Berkeley and Ross Taylor. Without their willingness to listen, to read and to criticise, this final text would have been immeasurably the poorer. At the same time, I want to put on record my gratitude to the many general practitioners, mainly but not entirely in the north-east of Scotland, who have contributed both time and thought in taking part in the various projects which illustrate this text.

Any research worker depends on his statistician and I am no exception. Ianthe Dingwall-Fordyce has helped me at many stages in the fieldwork described in this book and guided the planning and writing of the middle part of Chapter 12. Richard Morton and his staff in the Aberdeen University Department of Medical Illustration have also offered help beyond what is available to many attempting research and their contribution to the fifth of my illustrative projects was of particular importance.

Like most authors, I have come to depend on highly skilled secretarial support; the first half of the work was most capably seen into typescript by Mrs Rosemary Richardson and the remainder by Mrs Etta Duncan. To both, I would like to express my most sincere thanks.

Finally, three generations of my family have contributed to broadening my thinking about my work and have put up patiently with the consequences of what has followed; I hope that they will feel that this book makes their support seem to have been worth while.

John Howie
Aberdeen, 1979

FOREWORD

Among several recent major developments which characterise British general practice is its acceptance as a full university subject. In part this has been due to the growth of research thinking and research activity within health service practice but the acquisition of academic status has itself accelerated that process. There is evident now an increasing interest among family doctors in the whole scientific sequence summarised by the term 'research' and it is therefore timely that Dr Howie, a senior university lecturer, has written this book which so admirably explains how to initiate, design, execute, analyse and present a project, be it simple and small scale or more complex and substantial.

During a long academic career I have been fortunate in being able to assist a number of colleagues to make their debut in research, in both clinical and operational settings; and I have been further privileged to act as critic to those with more established research reputations. Such experience (tempered by a belief that my own researches should be subject to standards of scrutiny no less rigorous than those I apply to the work of others) has convinced me, firstly, that many more general practitioners could be useful researchers and secondly, that doctors who are guided into genuine scientific inquiry, however modest, are almost always in consequence more discriminating and fulfilled people.

Hitherto help with the creation or development of ideas has not been easily available to all those who are or could become interested in research in general practice. Dr Howie's book goes far towards meeting this existing need but will also, I am confident, help to generate new demand. He is well qualified to offer such assistance, having combined in his own career laboratory, clinical, teaching and research practice. I particularly like and commend his judicious use of personal research experience – including an honest account of why a project can fail. Dr Howie has successfully expressed his own enthusiasm for the research sequence and this essential vitality makes the book readable as well as informative – the author is proof of the belief that research should be enjoyable and not merely a chore to be done with an eye to its value in the career market.

It has been my privilege and pleasure to observe the conception and gestation of this monograph. Now that delivery has taken place into the capable hands of Croom Helm, I predict that *Research in*

Foreword

General Practice will become a thriving, significant and enduring contribution to the renaissance of general medical practice and family medicine.

I.M. Richardson
JP, MD, PhD, FRCP, FRCGP, DPH
James Mackenzie Professor of General Practice
University of Aberdeen

1 INTRODUCTION

Good research, thoughtfully planned and carefully carried out, is one of the most compelling and absorbing of the many professional activities open to the general practitioner. And 25,000 general practitioners and their aggregate of unanswered questions and untested impressions remain one of the most significant sources of research potential available to contemporary medicine.

Research is not a particularly difficult activity although it does require the ability to think clearly in an organised way. It need not require extensive knowledge of experimental or statistical techniques nor the possession of an extensive vocabulary or jargon. Simply defined it is the process of attempting to discover facts by critical investigation. Research is the essential basis for describing the work of any discipline, for testing the value of established practices and for assessing the importance of suggested advances. It is as relevant and necessary to general practice as to specialist medicine or surgery, obstetrics or pathology, or any other branch of medicine.

However, it would be wrong to regard research too lightly. Research has rules which must be followed, methods to be understood and applied and pitfalls to be avoided. Many of the rules for research in general practice are common to research in any field but there are specific problems relating to study of this particular area of clinical work and specific ways of tackling them. Some of the problems relate to the continuing debates as to whether general practice is an art or a science, whether it is related more closely to clinical medicine or to behavioural science and whether 'goodness' in general practice can be defined and measured. These difficulties reflect the importance of the doctor-patient relationship in the daily work of the general practitioner and its unique influence in the individual consultation.

Until recently relatively few general practitioners have been interested in research. The 1970 report of the British Medical Association Planning Unit estimated that a third of all general practitioners had participated in some research project during the previous three years, although this involvement had been mainly in trials designed by pharmaceutical companies. But now there are signs of an increase in the number of doctors participating in and designing research centred on the special problems and needs of general practice.

Much of this more recent involvement has been in projects organised by university departments, either of general practice or of other related disciplines, or in projects conceived by the Royal College of General Practitioners at national and local level. A recent review (The Nuffield Provincial Hospitals Trust, 1976) identified over 400 papers from general practice which had appeared in British medical or general practice journals during the five years up to 1975. If this figure seems impressive at first sight, it is nevertheless the starting point for stating my aims in writing this book.

Aims of This Book

To Encourage More Doctors to Initiate Their Own Research

It is hard to attend any meeting of general practitioners, educational or political, without realising the wide range of clinical and administrative problems in general practice which are waiting to be solved. Almost everyone has an opinion and often completely opposite points of view are argued without any evidence – other than personal impressions – to support them. An output of 400 research papers over five years from 25,000 general practitioners represents less than one completed project for every 300 doctors each year! This is a significant under-use of the discipline's undoubted capacity to contribute to understanding and developing the role of general practice in the maintenance of health and care of illness in our community. I believe that among the main reasons for this missed opportunity are a quite unnecessary fear of the unknown, and an unawareness that research is a fascinating and rewarding activity well within the abilities of most interested general practitioners.

To Improve the Research that is Done

Part of my work involves reading papers submitted to medical journals and theses presented for higher degrees. Another part involves helping doctors already doing research on their own or planning to start. It is sad how often interesting ideas and months of hard work end up frustrated because of avoidable weaknesses in design; or adequately designed studies fail to realise their potential because the originators do not assemble their findings to the best advantage, do not interpret their findings reasonably, or do not present them attractively. The second aim of this book is therefore to help doctors who are planning research or have already embarked on a project to make the fullest use of their opportunities and to avoid as many as possible of the errors which will either invalidate or reduce the value of their work.

To Contribute to Training for General Practice

All 'official' lists of objectives in training for general practice include a requirement that some teaching in research methods and their applications should be given. There are practical opportunities for trainee general practitioners to make contributions to their training practices by identifying and evaluating possible changes in practice routine. In addition, valuable prizes are now available for competition by trainees and younger principals, awards being made both for outlines of research proposals and for actual research done. At present any teaching in research that takes place is normally done on day-release schemes, but the best place to put theory to the test is in the training practice; this book aims to help both the trainer and the trainee who would like to make this objective more of a reality than it is at present.

To Help Develop Critical Thinking in General Practice

All advances in knowledge and improvements in practice depend on collecting information and interpreting it appropriately (research!). But too often general practitioners still quote their 'experience' based on far too few incidents to be capable of reasoned analysis, or accept at face value published research or advertising literature. Even a modest degree of familiarity with the process of research, with the specific problems of general practice research and with the common errors of research design, should encourage a substantial increase in the ability of general practitioners to defend themselves against the 'soft sell' image which they have tended to acquire in recent years.

To Demonstrate that Research is a Personal Activity

My last aim is more personal. I have always believed that research is not merely a technical process but reflects the personality, beliefs and hopes of the research worker. I hope through the pages of this book to portray research as a living activity, which adds to and is wholly compatible with the ideals and work of the general practitioner.

A Simple Research Framework

Any general practice consultation can be conducted or discussed at widely different levels of complexity. Commonly, and often reasonably, the presenting symptom or sign – usually physical, such as diarrhoea, rash or cough – is assessed and treated as an isolated complaint. At a deeper level, a physical complaint can be considered along with relevant psychological or social implications – the effect of recurrent lumbago on ability to earn; or the significance of an apparently simple breast lump to a patient whose mother has secondaries from breast cancer. And, at a third level, these physical, psychological and social features may require to be placed in a wider political context relating management to, for example, realities of limits and allocations of health service resources. No one approach is always right or always wrong. The ideal may not be realistic, and pressures, particularly those of time, may dictate the need for compromise. But in general the more intricate the problem presented by the patient, the more likely that greater skill in consultation will be called for and that greater professional knowledge and insight will be needed.

So it is with research. Simple questions are more easily answered than complex ones. In the same way that I have suggested thinking of consultations in three ways I find it helpful to think of research at three levels of difficulty. Each is appropriate for different purposes and all fall within the compass of the interested and thoughtful general practitioner. But beginners should normally start on relatively straightforward projects which can be elaborated as experience and confidence grow.

Level One

The simple diagrammatic representation of general practice as the intermediate part of Figure 1.1 is familiar to many.

Figure 1.1: Care of All Morbidity

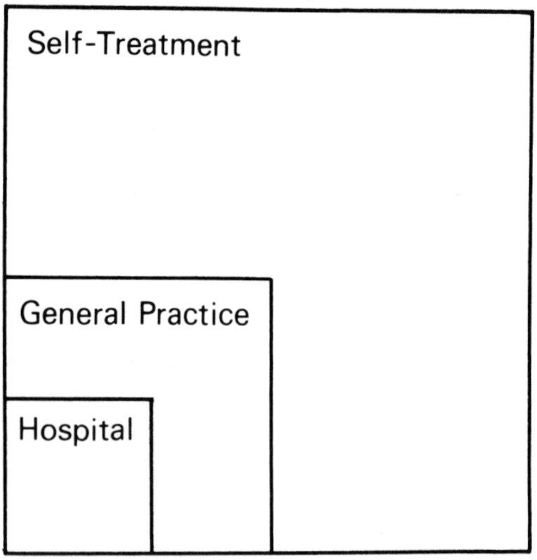

Self-Treatment

General Practice

Hospital

When this figure was reproduced by Fry in 1966 he suggested that three-quarters of all morbidity was cared for outside qualified medical care (by patients themselves, relatives, pharmacists' advice, advice from journals and radio) and one-quarter by doctors. Of the quarter seen by doctors, nine-tenths was seen in general practice alone and one-tenth reached hospital medicine. These proportions remain remarkably accurate today and this diagram acts as a useful starting point for identifying some of the problems and opportunities facing general practice research.

My 'first level' of research involves identifying single topics and examining them within the boundaries of the general practice setting. Table 1.1 lists some of the subjects which have been successfully studied in this way in recent years; Table 1.2 demonstrates how one of these (workload), which was initially examined in fairly general terms, has been examined subsequently to provide finer detail.

Neither Table 1.1 nor Table 1.2 does more than hint at the possibilities which abound. For instance, neither refers to simple clinical studies of those illnesses which are commonly seen in general practice and rarely seen elsewhere and Table 1.3 provides a small sample of useful, straightforward studies which have been carried out by family doctors working entirely within general practice.

Table 1.1: Examples of Single Topics for Study within Practice

Records	:	Dawes (1972)
Workload	:	Wright (1968)
Morbidity	:	Williams (1970)
Prescribing	:	Skegg *et al.* (1977)
Vocational Training	:	Freeman & Byrne (1976)
Investigation	:	Taylor *et al.* (1975)

Table 1.2: Examples of Further Studies on a Single Topic from Table 1.1 (Workload)

Certification	:	McDonald & McLean (1971)
Home Visits	:	Marsh *et al.* (1972)
Telephone Use	:	Reedy (1975)
Frequent Attenders	:	Courtenay *et al.* (1974)
Out-of-hours Work	:	Crowe *et al.* (1976)

Table 1.3: Examples of Clinical Studies Conducted Within General Practice

Diarrhoea	:	Everett (1973)
Barbiturate Prescribing	:	Wells (1973)
Blood Pressure	:	Hart (1970)
Bereavement	:	Rees (1971)
Cervical Screening	:	Scaife (1972)
Influenza	:	Taylor (1971)

This is the kind of research which forms the backbone of general practice investigation and there is much more still to be done.

Level Two

Instead of concentrating on single topics within the confines of general practice, my second level of research complexity covers studies which attempt to look in rather greater depth at relationships between topics of either clinical or behavioural type. I find it helpful to think of the three triangles shown in Figure 1.2.

The relationships or interactions outlined by these diagrams have been widely discussed but inadequately measured. Not enough is known about relationships between doctors and their patients and how these influence the presentation and management of illness. Again the complexities of relationships between the physical-psychological-social aspects of illness are accepted, but not well documented, and the different emphases given by different doctors to similar consultations is a major problem which has to be considered in any research project. The third interaction between clinical information-diagnosis-management is also an important one. Are, for example, histories taken

Figure 1.2: Some Related Features of General Practice

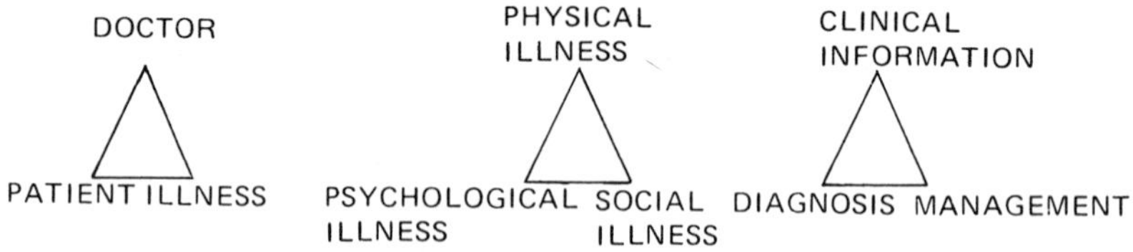

to justify or determine diagnostic or therapeutic decisions? These three triangles are only a few of many which can be visualised. Even the single subjects listed in Tables 1.1, 1.2 and 1.3 can be paired or grouped for deeper study. What, for example, is the relationship between workload and record keeping or between telephone use and home visiting rates?

Research at this depth will more often require – or naturally lead to – several linked studies before producing the results hoped for, and is particularly suited to producing a thesis for a higher degree.

Level Three

Both of the previous levels have kept within the confines of general practice. For my third level I would like to return to my original diagram (Figure 1.1) and add two pairs of arrows to it as in Figure 1.3.

Are the lines separating the three zones of the figure boundaries or barriers between parts of the system of health care? How is the management of patients in general practice influenced by the relationships between specialists and general practitioners, or between general practitioners and their nursing and social work colleagues? What are the implications of the availability and standing of local specialist services to patients deciding whether to self-treat or consult their

Figure 1.3: Boundaries or Barriers?

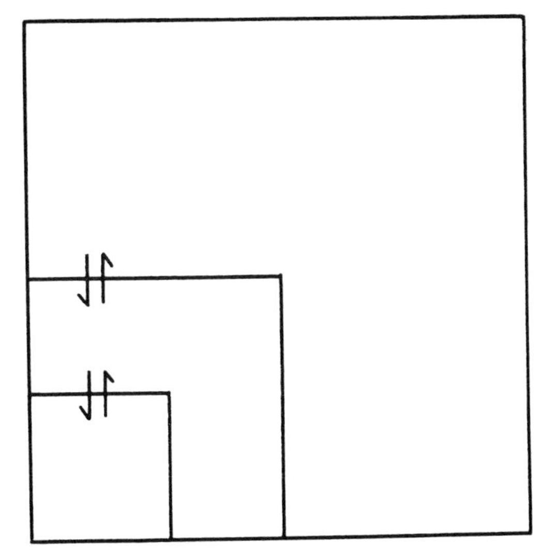

family doctor and on the treatment he provides? How effectively do doctors in practice interpret their patients' illnesses to the consultants to whom they refer?

Research into these broader issues produces substantial difficulties in design and calls for an understanding of spheres of work other than one's own. A team approach is often needed and this produces special problems which will be discussed later. If general practice research often needs the point of view of the specialist or social scientist, the reverse is equally true. General practice research has a contribution to make to research in other fields; for the contribution to be effective it must, however, be a thoroughly professional one.

Recent Research Trends

It is true that the general practice research projects which have attracted most publicity in recent years have been those organised on the largest scale, supported by the most substantial funding and backed by the greatest expertise in organisation. The Royal College of General Practitioners' Oral Contraceptive Study (RCGP, 1974) has been a model of operational efficiency; the second National Morbidity Study (jointly sponsored by the Department of Health and Social Security, the Office of Population Censuses and Surveys and the Royal College of General Practitioners) has produced much valuable information on the work of general practice, albeit at a surface level (OPCS, 1974) and the Manchester University department's assessments of vocational training for general practice represent many years of painstaking study incorporating a major specialist educational contribution (Freeman & Byrne, 1976).

Important and necessary though such major and collaborative undertakings are, the combined published work from RCGP Research Units and Faculties and from university departments represents in numerical terms only a small proportion of papers published from general practice. Most originate from service practices and most require little or no outside financial support.

It is interesting to look briefly at the principal themes covered in the 400 papers referred to on page 12. Drug trials were reported in 89 studies and 67 papers described an aspect of the natural history of illness as seen in general practice. A further 66 papers assessed forms of management other than drug trials, 56 described aspects of practice organisation or the use of hospitals, 34 described activities in the fields of preventive medicine, screening or health education and 30 studied the processes by which decisions on diagnosis and management are made.

On the other hand, the total of studies devoted to education in its various aspects, the behaviour of patients, prescribing, record keeping, morbidity and workload, the concept of team care and the relationships between doctors and patients, came to only around 100 in the five-year period surveyed. By the time this book is published, these patterns may have changed. Studies on prescribing are increasing, for example, while those on workload and morbidity are becoming less common. Many challenges and opportunities clearly remain.

This Book

The process of research starts with asking questions and ends with publishing results. Each step depends on the one before and should be influenced by anticipation of later stages of the process. The complete process falls into four recognisable parts and this book devotes one section to each. Part one follows the process from the asking of questions, through developing the idea, reading the relevant literature, to producing either a hypothesis for testing or a statement of objectives for the study. The second part discusses the design of studies, their financing and the organisation of the fieldwork. The third part looks at the analysis and interpretation of results and the fourth part covers the presentation of findings.

Perhaps my greatest difficulty has been deciding how to balance discussion of the principles of research (the do's and dont's) with illustrations of what these mean and imply. From time to time in the text I will refer to good examples from the literature of general practice; but from my own experience I know just how many problems and difficulties a tidily presented paper may play down or simply exclude from consideration, and also how unfair it may be to criticise design or presentation without knowledge of relevant background information, perhaps omitted from the report in the cause of brevity. Instead of risking unfair criticism of the attempts of others to do research, I have chosen to describe in some detail six projects in which I have had a major personal involvement. These descriptions will tell of what failed as well as what worked, of the frustrations as well as the pleasures, of problems created by ignoring the advice I now give others, and of the occasions where good luck has compensated for guesswork or opportunism has allowed mistakes to appear successes.

The six projects include two clinical trials, one of which was successful and one unsuccessful, a multi-doctor questionnaire study, an attempt to assess an apparent improvement in communication between hospital and general practice, a study based on existing practice records and an experiment in the use of photography to aid definition of the way in which general practitioners prescribe. The projects will be described as they evolved in three separate chapters, one at the end of each of the first three sections. I hope that in these chapters the more personal implications of research will provide the reader with a proper balance between the ideal and the real.

References

British Medical Association, 'Primary Medical Care', *Planning Unit Report*, no.4 (BMA, London, 1970).

Courtenay, M.J.F., Curwen, M.P., Dawe, D., Robinson, J. & Stern, M.J., 'Frequent Attenders in a Family Practice', *Journal of the Royal College of General Practitioners*, 24 (1974), pp.251-61.

Crowe, M.G.F., Hurwood, D.S. & Taylor, R.W., 'Out-of-hours Calls in a Leicestershire Practice', *British Medical Journal*, 1 (1976), pp.1582-4.

Dawes, K.S., 'Survey of General Practice Records', *British Medical Journal*, 3 (1972), pp.219-23.

Everett, M.T., 'The Place of Antibiotics in the Treatment of Acute Gastro-enteritis in General Practice: a Controlled Trial', *Journal of the Royal College of General Practitioners*, 23 (1973), pp.183-93.

Freeman, J. & Byrne, P.S., 'The Assessment of Vocational Training for General Practice', *Reports from General Practice*, no.17 (Royal College of General Practitioners, London, 1976).

Fry, J., *Profiles of Disease* (E. & S. Livingstone, London & Edinburgh, 1966, p.9).

Hart, J.T., 'Semicontinuous Screening of a Whole Community for Hypertension', *Lancet*, 2 (1970), pp.223-6.

McDonald, A. & McLean, I.G., 'Study of the Work of General Practitioners', *Practitioner*, 207 (1971), pp.680-8.

Marsh, G.N., McNay, R.A. & Whewell, J., 'Survey of Home Visiting by General Practitioners in North-east England', *British Medical Journal*, 1 (1972), pp.487-92.

Nuffield Provincial Hospitals Trust, 'General Practice Research', unpublished papers of Symposium, 1976.

Office of Population Censuses and Surveys, 'Morbidity Statistics from General Practice', *Studies on Medical and Population Subjects*, no.26 (HMSO, London, 1974).

Reedy, B.L.E.C., 'Telephone Messages Received by Seven General Practices', *Journal of the Royal College of General Practitioners*, 25 (1975), pp.916-23.

Rees, W.D., 'The Hallucinations of Widowhood', *British Medical Journal*, 4 (1971), pp.37-41.

Royal College of General Practitioners, *Oral Contraceptives and Health* (Whitefriars Press, London, 1974).

Scaife, B., 'Survey of Cervical Cytology in General Practice', *British Medical Journal*, 3 (1972), pp.200-2.

Skegg, D.C.G., Doll, R. & Perry, J., 'Use of Medicines in General Practice', *British Medical Journal*, 1 (1977), pp.1561-3.

Taylor, M.P., 'Influenza 1969-70', *Journal of the Royal College of General Practitioners*, 21 (1971), pp.17-22.

Taylor, R.J., Howie, J.G.R., Brodie, J. & Porter, I.A., 'Use of Bacteriological

Investigations by General Practitioners', *British Medical Journal*, 3 (1975), pp.635-6.
Wells, F.O., 'Prescribing Barbiturates: Drug Substitution in General Practice', *Journal of the Royal College of General Practitioners*, 23 (1973), pp.164-7.
Williams, W.O., 'A Study of General Practitioners' Workload in South Wales 1965-6', *Reports from General Practice*, no.12 (Royal College of General Practitioners, London, 1970).
Wright, H.J., 'General Practice in South-west England', *Reports from General Practice*, no.8 (Royal College of General Practitioners, London, 1968).

PART ONE

THINKING ABOUT RESEARCH

2 ASKING QUESTIONS

This apparently simple activity merits a chapter of its own for two reasons. First, it represents the initial step in the research process; without a good question useful research will not develop. Many doctors who would like to try a piece of research fail to get started, not because they lack ability to ask questions but because they do not know how to translate the problems and frustrations or the successes and pleasures of their working lives into the kind of questions which will lead to worthwhile research. Second, and in contrast, it is possible to make the mistake of asking questions which are too difficult to answer or not important enough to merit the necessary outlays of time and resources. I want to look briefly at these complementary problems.

Recognising Questions

Almost any part of the general practitioner's working life can provide a starting point for research. From activities as diverse as, for example, visiting in the home or consulting in the surgery, signing certificates or writing referral letters, doing emergency night calls, prescribing, choosing what to carry in the medical bag or on which day to have the still traditional half-day off, problems can be identified, inconsistencies noticed and questions asked. Why does Mrs S always phone for a visit on Monday mornings? What are the characteristics of patients who request visits and do these differ on the different days of the week? What kind of problems are presented to deputising doctors and how do these differ from those presented out-of-hours to the 'regular' doctor. Dr C always seems busier with home visits on Monday morning than Drs A and B. Do some partners attract more requests for home visits or out-of-hours work than others?

Or, why is my Monday evening surgery so much more chaotic than my senior partner's? How does he always seem to keep pace with his appointment list while I fall behind although I have fewer patients booked? He does seem to see a lot of older patients – are they all 'return' appointments while I see all the 'new' patients? Perhaps he is better with the old patients and probably I cope better with the children because my own family is young – but maybe it's the other way round and the old patients don't really like seeing a new doctor. Perhaps it would be better if the third partner did the other Monday evening surgery. . .

Or, did that little girl with the cough and the runny nose have measles or was it just a cold? Does the measles vaccine really work? Will the cough mixture I prescribed help? I know that people say these mixtures are useless but I always use them for my own children. Or is it because I prescribe them that so many patients with colds come to see me? Was that last patient given valium because I was in a hurry and should I have asked her back for a longer chat? If I really thought her headache was due to tension why did I agree with her that she had migraine? What is migraine – and do any of these treatments really work?

Or, why does Mr J always come to get his ears syringed when I'm busy? Why does he get so much wax? Maybe it would be easier to ask the nurse to syringe the ears as they do in the practice down the road. Do these wax softeners really help? The rep says they do and his graphs looked impressive. But I don't really know what to believe about the studies these chaps produce. Maybe when Dr Y retires we should go for a full-time nurse rather than another doctor with the population falling because of rehousing. And, what other implications does the rehousing have on our practice, administratively and clinically?

It is not only during the working day in the practice that the interesting or unexpected may turn up. Experience, for example, in a part-time industrial medical job, or while visiting a patient in hospital, or even while attending a committee meeting may spark a question about one's own particular methods of working or about clinical or administrative practice in more general terms. Snatches of overheard conversations; items in the press or on radio or television; comments made on social occasions by friends or acquaintances; articles read in journals or in advertisements: any of these may surprise or puzzle, or irritate and annoy. These are the sources of questions about our work, and it is these questions which will provide the basis for our research.

Good and Bad Questions

Although the potential for asking questions is almost without limit, not all questions make good research questions. And what might be a good research question for a doctor working in one setting might be a quite unsatisfactory question for a doctor working in a different situation.

The first essential of a good question is that it is *important* enough to be worth answering. Importance may relate to the seriousness of the topic (the side effects of immunisation or of drugs such as oral contraceptives) or to the frequency with which it happens (writing certificates, home visits, prescribing for diarrhoea). Importance may be specific to a single doctor (his own workload), to a practice (how many receptionists to employ), to a group of practices (a policy on anorectic drugs) or more widely applicable. A question may also be important because, although relating neither to serious illness nor to a common activity, it establishes a principle with wider implications. An example of this last qualification was our Aberdeen study of use of the bacteriology services by local general practitioners (Taylor *et al.*, 1975). Previous studies of laboratory use had identified doctors as high or low users of laboratory services as if these qualities were applicable to laboratory use generally. We believed, and showed, that a high user of one test (say throat swabs) might be a low user of another (say urine culture) and that many doctors were in fact very selective high users of the laboratory. This study has implications for evaluation of other specialist services as referral habits may again be much more selective than is sometimes assumed. At this still early stage in the definition of both the content of general practice work and of the way in which different doctors approach similar problems this justification for doing research is particularly valid.

The second criterion of a good question is that it should be an *interesting* one – not as unnecessary a qualification as it might at first seem to be. This is important if helpers are required either from amongst one's own colleagues in practice or from 'outside' sources, including specialists, laboratory workers and statisticians. What interests one person does not necessarily interest another; research may fail to reach a successful conclusion because an enthusiast has overestimated the general attractiveness of his proposals. In addition, even the most committed research worker may find his own interest in a study difficult to maintain over a complete project and I will refer to this again shortly.

The third credential of a good question is that it is *answerable.* The cause of breast cancer, the indications for treatment in hypertension, the aetiology of multiple sclerosis and the many other questions of this type are both important and interesting. However, except in unusual circumstances which would almost certainly imply major support from government or equivalent research funds, it is unrealistic to expect them to be answered by research initiated in general practice by general practitioners. The criteria of realistic research will become apparent in later chapters.

The issue of time is important. Motivation can last about three to four years for those developing an interest of their own, but rarely more than a year (and often an 'academic' year – October to May – at that) for those recruited to help. In addition, as time passes, the original criteria of selection and measurement may tend to change in a slight but cumulative and thus important way, the original need for the study may become less pressing and, again because motivation is not easily maintained, variable and unpredictable losses of quality in the information available may spoil earlier work of good quality. For these reasons long-term research is particularly difficult to design and interpret and the beginner in research should probably start with a piece of research which can be completed within a relatively short time.

In summary, good research questions are:

important questions – personally, locally or more generally;
interesting questions; and
questions which are capable of being answered and answered preferably within a predictable and relatively short period of time.

Bad research questions are those the solutions of which is beyond the resources of the research worker.

Good scientists, according to Medawar, study the most important problems they think they can solve!

Selecting a Question

Uncertainty is a reality the general practitioner has to come to terms with to survive his daily work. For both his own and his patients' benefit he is required to accept in good faith much that is unproven or in practical terms unprovable. Maybe he questions too little. On the other hand, the research worker may seem to question too much – about diagnosis and treatment, about patients and illnesses, about knowledge, techniques of practice and attitudes. A balance has to be found.

My own practice is to make notes of the questions I ask myself on any piece of paper handy at the time – an EC10 in the surgery, a note on a telephone pad, or an envelope in my pocket. If, after a day or two, the question still seems to qualify as a possible 'good' research question I add it to a list on my office wall. Once or twice a year I revise this list, discarding questions which have grown less attractive as time passes and those which fuller enquiry has shown to have been adequately answered elsewhere (but don't be afraid to repeat previous work – different results are often produced). Often it is possible to see that several questions are challenging the same principle and indeed recognition of this may be the first stage of the development of a research question into a research idea – the subject of the next chapter. After this process of revising and discarding, the questions which are left are likely to be those which genuinely interest and seem important. They next need to be explored and developed further. By now the construction of a viable research project is a distinct possibility.

3 FORMING IDEAS

Having found a question which seems interesting, important and solvable, it is time to think in general terms about possible ways of answering it. I want to start this short chapter by discussing three principles which should guide all research planning.

Three Principles

Take Time

If a good question has been asked, the temptation to hurry to answer it is understandable – but dangerous. Rushing through the preliminary stages more often than not leads to disappointment later when it becomes clear that major flaws have led to the wrong information being collected, often badly and in a manner which means the information can be neither analysed nor interpreted. If enough time and trouble is taken in the early stages of research, then those problems which do turn up after the project has begun should be of a relatively minor nature suitable for on-the-spot solution. The fear of being beaten to the finishing post is almost always less real than the risk of falling into the water jump.

At this stage, predict what the answer to your question might be and estimate what results you would need to collect to support your prediction. Will new information be required, or can existing records be used? Although the stepwise progression through the research sequence as outlined in Chapter 1 will require to be followed fairly closely once the research idea has become firm, at this stage considerable flexibility of thinking is not only justifiable but is to be encouraged. Visualise your paper appearing in print, the MD thesis you are going to write, the audience you will address. What will catch interest and hold attention? Make some notes; write them into a short statement of aims and plans, then put this away and leave it for a few weeks or until after the holidays or after Christmas. Then go over the process again. Be willing to remould your original question and developing idea to fit the time and resources which you expect to have available or hope to find. A good project will probably take about twelve months to develop from the stage of asking the question to making any necessary application for funds or starting to collect results. An experienced worker may require less time but usually this is because the field of study is already familiar to him. Many good projects take even longer to think through to their apparent starting point.

Aim for Perfection

Throughout this book the need for compromise between the possible and the ideal is a recurring theme. In research it is often necessary to settle for second best because the ideal is not attainable but too often third best or worse is more tempting and is accepted. The 'he's only a general practitioner' attitude of journals and referees and of grant-giving bodies still prevails in some quarters although fortunately it is diminishing. Nothing does a greater disservice to general practice and to the concept of research in general practice than poorly conceived and poorly carried out research. Have nothing to do with it. Remember that *modest* research and *poor* research are not the same. Aim to design a project that provides valid even if relatively simple findings and avoid being involved with any study which seems based on weak or inadequate planning no matter how superficially attractive it may seem. The simple and valid study is the basis of progress; weakly conceived research retards it.

Think for Yourself

The compressed undergraduate curriculum of most medical schools leaves students too little time to think for themselves and provides a far from ideal background for research thinking. Early postgraduate training, now increasingly geared to passing factually based diploma examinations, does little to remedy this weakness of modern medical education. Start the attempt to explain or solve your research problem by stating honestly to yourself what *you* think the possible or probable answers to your own question to be. Be willing to make any suggestion which you believe to be true even if it contradicts the most fundamental 'rules' of traditional medical teaching, challenges the view of eminent clinicians or teachers, or differs from the views of textbooks (views which, incidentally, often seem to be passed unchallenged and unauthenticated from generation to generation). Back your personal hunch or judgement as to which is the better treatment, as to what might be the cause of this disease or that syndrome, or the reason for this problem or for that success or whatever.

From the moment that someone else influences your thinking about the best way to find an answer to a question, it becomes that much less likely that you will be able to plan independently of his advice or ideas and that much more likely that your subsequent efforts will be along traditional lines, the shortcomings of which may have already contributed to your question arising. Although an experienced research thinker will almost reflexly disagree with any suggestion offered (at least at first) the inexperienced research worker may find this difficult to do. An additional difficulty may lie not in being able to have a *very* different idea to someone else's, but in being able to have a *slightly* different idea. Just as the Western ear is tuned to the musical frequencies of tones and semitones and finds the finer differences of Eastern music difficult to utilise, so also the mind of the inexperienced research worker is tuned to the familiar rather than the unfamiliar.

The difficulty of thinking in an original way is described splendidly by de Bono in his classic book *The Use of Lateral Thinking*. (This short and eminently readable book is worthwhile for any research worker.) His argument is developed in this way: if someone were asked to describe the Figures 3.1 and 3.2 below, the range of answers would be predictable and basically unimaginative. Figure 3.1 would be described as, for example, four squares made into a fifth square, or a box including a cross, or six equal lines each in contact with two or three others, and so on. Figure 3.2 would be described either as a capital H or as a set of rugby posts but not much else.

If, however, Figure 3.1 is redrawn as Figure 3.3, the original square can be seen to be composed of four Ts. Now that the concept of building with Ts has been introduced Figure 3.2 is readily recognised as comprising two Ts and in retrospect it is hard to see how this could ever have been missed.

Figure 3.1:

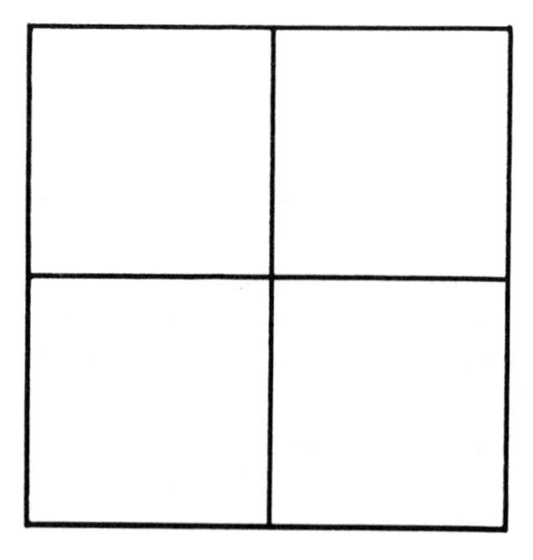

Figure 3.2:

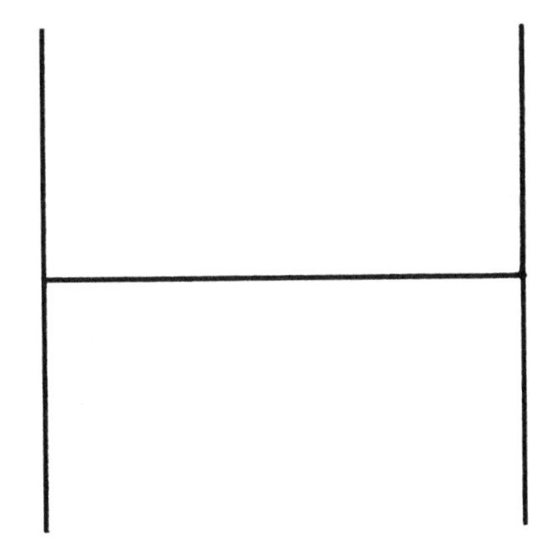

Figure 3.3:

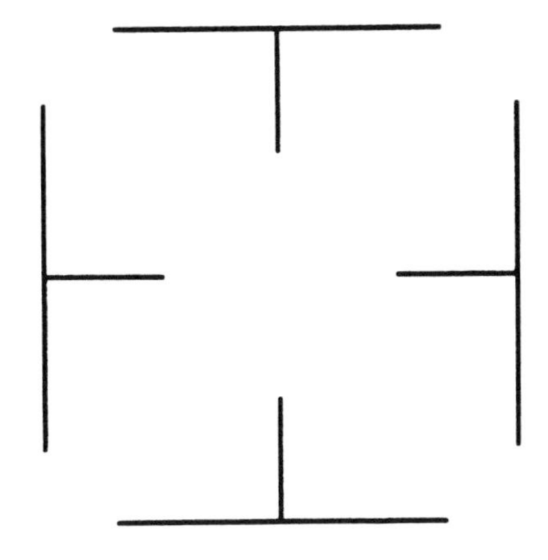

Equally, now that the mind is thinking in terms of Ts rather than straight lines, it is unlikely that Figure 3.2 would be described as six Is, although each T could be equally well thought of as three adjoining Is.

My concern is that originality is not only a positive attribute but is also the absence of the negative attribute of conditioned thinking. Try first, therefore, to develop the idea to help answer your question from your own insights into the problem which interests you. It is from this position that you will be best able to benefit from the advice you should now seek from other sources.

Consulting Colleagues

The value of consulting friends and colleagues in the early stages of a research interest is as real as it must seem obvious. However, too much consultation can be as unhelpful as too little. Be influenced by the opinions you receive but do not allow yourself to be dominated by them. Ask people with a reputation for being critical; if you can find people who are known to be constructive as well, that is an added bonus. Leaving aside discussion with those who have technical help to offer (for example statisticians, data processors and colleagues able to provide essential technical assistance – their important and essential contributions are discussed later) three opinions are probably worth seeking. Speak to someone with experience of general practice research – possibly someone in a university department of general practice. Speak to a general practitioner whose main job is service practice but who has a positive view of the need to keep an open but sceptical mind towards new developments. And, speak to someone you respect from outside general practice but who you think may be interested in the broader aspects of medical progress: a consultant in a specialist field, a friend working in a research unit, a colleague from a discipline related to medicine such as sociology or physiology. If you choose well, you will both be impressed by and benefit from the often remarkable breadth of vision and interest which apparently specialised research workers acquire from their work.

Reading the Literature

There is no debate about the need to read relevant literature and the next chapter provides advice on how to set about doing this. The question of when to carry out this often considerable undertaking is more open. In the same way that the views and advice of colleagues affect the way in which research is conceived, what is read can have a substantial influence either by broadening or by focusing thinking. It would obviously be wrong to suggest that reading should be confined to any one stage of developing a research idea; but the ordering of the sub-headings in this chapter reflects my own view of the priority which offers the greatest benefit.

Thinking Flexibly

From time to time during this period of thinking, discussing and reading about the question asked, it is useful to think back to the criteria of a good question. Is your original question still of interest, does it still seem important and what chance does there seem to be of finding an answer? Does the question you asked stand on its own or is it part of a more general theme which could be more easily tackled from a different starting point? For example, the original question 'How often do patients with abdominal pain want to discuss a personal problem?' might reflect an interest in the more general theme of 'How do patients wanting to discuss personal problems present them?' Abdominal pain may not be the best starting point if the real interest is in personal problems rather than abdominal pain. A new and possibly more rewarding question might be constructed along the lines 'Do patients with gynaecological symptoms usually wish to discuss personal problems?' In other words, is the question you are asking really the question you want to answer?

It is often here that advice from colleagues is most helpful. Although it is almost certainly true that the best time for original research is when the mind is young and active, age and experience bring a capacity to develop the ideas of others in a way which can change the direction of developing research enough to convert probable failure to probable success. Those asked for advice in the early stages of research planning almost always suggest further discussions after more time has been taken for reading and thinking; offers of this kind are meant and should be taken up.

The process of forming viable research ideas is a gradual one. Generalisations are slowly made more specific. The scope of the possible project becomes more sharply defined. Difficulties are anticipated and outcomes forecast. Realism replaces idealism. If at this stage the question you asked still interests you and still seems important, keep going. It is not yet necessary to commit yourself either to the format of the research or to the final wording of the question.

Reference

de Bono, E., *The Use of Lateral Thinking* (Cape, London, 1976).

4 READING THE LITERATURE

Many general practitioners have difficulty finding time to read medical literature either widely or regularly. Deciding how much of the time available should be allotted to reading medical newspapers, how much to journals about general practice, and how much to topics of more general medical interest is a further problem. However, what is read is mainly received by post and easily accessible. The doctor with a research interest has to face two extra problems; he has to find more time to read in depth on the subject of his choice and now has to search out what he needs rather than simply filter what he is offered.

Although all would agree that reading is an important part of the early stages of research there are different views on how much should be done and when it should be done. Some read early to determine what course their research should follow and others, of whom I am one, read later to check that a developing idea is on reasonable lines. The advantage of the first approach is that reading is undertaken with an open mind and the risks of repeating previous work are reduced; the advantage of the second approach is that it reduces the risk of being 'conditioned' by what others have done and led away from an original and personal line of thought. Both schools would agree that too much reading may become a distraction from actually doing research and that too little reading may unnecessarily limit the investigator's ability to make a useful contribution to his chosen field. Both schools would also agree that although reading should normally guide the research worker towards making a new contribution to his subject, it may sometimes be justifiable to repeat work already reported especially if the method of the previous study seems suspect or the results surprising.

This chapter discusses several complementary ways of searching the literature. 'Exploratory reading' covers the simple preliminary review essential for any research project and allows for the limited time and possibly limited facilities available to general practitioners trying to combine research and service work. Exploratory reading should be a part of the early stages of developing a research idea and will usually precede or immediately follow preliminary discussions of the idea with any colleagues who have been approached for advice. 'Comprehensive reading' discusses the methods of obtaining a wider cover of the literature and might be regarded as an optional, though desirable, extra.

The chapter ends with some advice on making reference lists and reference files.

Exploratory Reading

My first recommendation is to start simply and to extend the scope of the review if early results are encouraging. The *Journal of the Royal College of General Practitioners* (JRCGP) usually forms my own starting point for a search of general practice literature. Take the most recent year's bound volume available (or the equivalent in loose monthly journals together with the index) and turn to the index which will be found at either the back or the front of the volume. The JRCGP index lists references under both author and topic and, when there are several authors, lists each author separately. Start with the subject heading. If, for example, the theme being reviewed is 'workload', check this heading first; then identify possible headings for cross-references or related references. In a review of literature on workload these could include 'home visits', 'night visits' and 'practice organisation'. Depending on the particular interest being explored, other headings such as 'repeat prescribing' and 'telephone – use of' or alternatively 'morbidity' or 'immigrant populations' might also be of interest. Depending on the number of references this first check produces, repeat the exercise for the previous year. Be willing to go back about five years to begin with and aim to collect between a dozen and twenty references.

Then take these four or five volumes to a quiet part of the library – or home if lending rules allow – and look up and read the references carefully. Make notes on postcards or on a loose-leaf pad. Note the authors' names and where the work was done; make a judgement on the quality of the work, on its usefulness and on its relevance to your own idea; would the method used fit your opportunities? Could you develop the idea reported further? Do you believe the results reported? Do you agree with the interpretation of the results? Has the discussion missed an important point? And finally, note the references quoted.

In this way your list of references will mount quickly. Don't feel guilty at building on someone else's efforts – that is part of the healthy chain reaction of research and progress. Within an hour or two or an evening or two it should be possible to answer a few basic questions about your own embryo project. Has a lot already been done and published in this field of interest? Does early reading suggest a viable research idea which could make a contribution to knowledge and understanding? Are there any references which keep reappearing in the reference lists in other papers? Are there any authors who appear to have made large contributions to published work in this field? Are there any good review articles on the list? Although a review does not absolve the reader from reading the articles which have been quoted, for himself, it inevitably saves much time searching for references. If the review is good enough, it may be justifiable to assume that no important omissions will have occurred, but even in the best review, this always remains a possibility.

Amongst examples of valuable reviews published in recent years in the JRCGP are those by Green (1973) on the use of the laboratory, Elliot and Stevenson (1973) on the care of the elderly and Taylor (1977) on prescribing in general practice. Besides the JRCGP, the RCGP publication *Trends in General Practice* (1977) carries useful reviews of, for example, the general practitioner and the hospital (Louden) and the health team (Reedy).

As well as review articles, relevant editorial or leading articles should be looked for. This type of article may again be of particular value because it has been written by someone with wide experience in the particular field; leading articles often attempt to evaluate as well as list published work, and try to read into the future as well as survey the past.

The next stage is to turn again to the index page, this time to see if those who appear to be key authors have written other useful papers which cross-reference checking may have missed. Cryptic titles may have been used which defy allocation in a subject index – a hazard to be guarded against by writers as well as readers! Pursuing the example of a review of 'workload' a little further, repeated references will be found to publications by Marsh, Wright and Williams. Once again review of these articles and their reference lists would point backwards to an earlier key reference article in the field of workload study – that by Lees & Cooper (1963).

At this stage a decision has to be taken as to how far to look back into the past. Even if many apparently out-of-date references do lack relevance to planning new research, on many occasions a glance at a paper from an earlier decade can give a most interesting insight into what were seen as problems at that time and may add a useful perspective to the developing idea. The 1952 paper of Dunlop, Henderson and Inch in the field of general practice prescribing is one example of the lasting value of good original research.

By this time it is probable that a number of references will have been made to articles in journals other than that being used for the first stage of the search. The next step is to follow up the more accessible of these references, if possible choosing to read those more likely to help before those less likely to help. Journals become associated with a particular type and quality of article. The *Lancet* carries few reports from general practice, but usually good ones. The better of the less specialised of general practice research papers tend to appear in the *British Medical Journal* or JRCGP (and probably in that order) whereas the longer, more specialised or more philosophical general practice papers seem to reverse that priority. *Update* and the *Practitioner* concentrate on educational rather than original work and research papers appearing in these journals are often modified versions of papers declined – although not necessarily wisely – by the journals already mentioned. Papers appearing in journals outside this range, unless widely quoted, should usually be omitted until attempting a more comprehensive review at a later stage.

Then finally, repeat the search of the indexes of the journals referred to above (*British Medical Journal, Update, Practitioner* and *Lancet*), again following up new leads which seem promising. Remember that some journals, although none of those referred to above, index authors and subjects in separate catalogues. Also remember that correspondence columns often contain important comments and criticisms of more formal articles and should not be disregarded in any search of literature.

Watch for three things: beware of abstracts and quoting from these without checking the original article; beware of quoting other writers' quotations without first checking their accuracy and original context; and beware of quoting authors' conclusions as facts. In other words, make it a policy to read everything which is to be used as a reference in its original form whenever possible.

(This section assumes that the doctor has reasonably easy access to a modest postgraduate or undergraduate medical library; for doctors in more remote areas a number of alternative services are available and these are described shortly.)

Comprehensive Reading

After discussing the initial review with a friend or colleague and confirming that the developing idea is worth expanding, a number of further steps are advisable. First, of course, the references already collected may be followed more widely, with the review extending to the now considerable range of specialist journals available and to journals published in other countries. This may be of interest and value in suggesting direction and design of the developing project but equally may be time consuming and frustrating if references are in journals not stocked in the library being used. When problems of this kind arise it may be possible to borrow through the inter-library loan facilities which are now widely available or to enlist the assistance of the RCGP librarian as discussed below.

The second guide to a more extensive coverage of literature is the use of an indexing system of which the *Index Medicus* is the best-known example. This aid is available in most average-sized general libraries and any librarian will guide the new reader on its use. In this publication all material published in the world's medical literature is indexed by subject (including cross-references where possible) and by author much as in a single journal. Papers published in English are catalogued separately from those in foreign languages. Monthly editions are aggregated annually into the *Cumulative Index Medicus* which appears in separate subject and author editions. There tends to be repetition of references in the monthly editions, most but not all of which disappears in the annual editions. The comprehensiveness of this index is, of course, again limited by the suitability of titles for indexing. References may appear up to two years after their original date of publication.

A further method, painstaking but often rewarding, involves searching for articles which may have been missed because of the use of cryptic or inappropriate titles. An article on prescribing can, for example, discuss subjects as diverse as workload, communication, practice organisation, patient behaviour and so on without its being classified under any of these heads. There is no short cut to finding such articles. The only solution is to scan or read the summaries of all articles in whatever journals are selected. Surprisingly interesting and helpful results can come from this exercise, giving both breadth and depth to the more obvious reading already described. Clearly a limit has to be set on such an exercise both in terms of the number of years to review and the number of journals to cover – probably not more than five years and probably only the JRCGP and the 'Medical Practice' section of the *British Medical Journal.*

Lastly, in this section mention has to be made of material contained in reports (for example, from Royal Commissions or Health Department working parties), in monographs on the subject being studied and in textbooks. It is probable that important sources of this kind of information will have been identified in the reference lists of papers already read in the earlier stages of the review. References of this kind are more likely to be of conceptual than factual assistance as most important research work will have been published, at some stage, in article format.

Reviewing Services

A number of services are available to general practitioners who either do not wish to carry out a review for themselves or cannot because of inaccessibility of library services. The most useful of these are provided by the RCGP and are available through the librarian. A review of new general practice literature is prepared annually and reference lists on selected topics (audit, workload, night calls, the nurse, for example) are already available. New reviews of references on specific topics will be provided on request and a photocopying service which is available to all general practitioners will supplement this by reproducing complete articles where feasible. (Photocopying is, of course, expensive; the RCGP service is offered free to members up to a limited number of pages per annum. Non-members pay a small charge per page copied.) The College reference lists are, like any others, limited by the accuracy and completeness of the sources from which they are compiled and should normally be seen as complementing rather than replacing the personal efforts advised earlier in this section.

A number of commercial abstracting and indexing services (for example MEDLARS – Medical Literature and Retrieval Service) do exist, but these are expensive to subscribe to and provide information more helpful to specialist than to general practice research.

Collecting References

It is often helpful if information gained from specific searching or general reading can be retained in a usable manner. Some people have a great capacity to recall what they have read without making notes or using reference systems. But most of us need a more formal and more reliable system of recall.

Various techniques are advocated. Some readers photocopy avidly while others tear out articles with equal enthusiasm; the first policy is expensive when done on a large scale, the second only possible when the journal is your own. Some keep annotated contents pages, others store annual journal index lists. Some make notes on postcards and file the postcards. When reviewing literature for a specific project my own policy is a combination of these approaches. Most material from journals can be summarised on 8 in. x 6 in. postcards, noting all authors and the exact reference (pages, volume, year, title and journal name). The key information, including a comment on its context and the author's and my own interpretation of its validity and importance, is noted below the reference heading. Although leading articles and review articles may be dealt with in the same way, some which are difficult to summarise or include useful reference lists are photocopied or torn out. A reference from a textbook may be noted on a postcard or photocopied. A photocopy may be justified if the extract is a long one or if the book has been borrowed from a distant source – noting, of course, that copyright restrictions may exist in relation to the use of such material. A government memorandum may be retained complete; a drug advertisement may be kept with a circle round the key statement. I use a headed file in which all relevant cards, photocopies and tear-outs are stored. At the start of my search I list all the sources to be checked on the flap of the folder and tick these off as I progress through the list.

When reading more generally I note only those occasional references which either seem of unusual interest or which appear to offer potential as starting material for new projects. The general material sits on a slowly growing single pile of reprints, journals, abstracts and postcards now several inches high which I often look through when developing new research ideas. This collection is weeded out rather less frequently than it should be, some gaining promotion to the 'research question list' I described at the end of Chapter 2, but rather more suffering relegation to the waste-paper bucket because its attractiveness has failed to stand the test of time. My research files stay thin enough to be useful but thick enough to be able to recognise quickly the best available short-cut to a more detailed search of literature when this becomes necessary.

It is worth remembering that one's general reading can help research not only by stimulating new ideas or by changing or confirming the direction in which a current idea or project is developing, but sometimes by providing a stimulus to 'write up' some findings which have been left unreported for some reason. It is, of course, unrealistic to hope to read everything that comes to hand from government articles to advertising literature. My own policy is to read regularly most leading articles and a few selected articles from one general practice journal (the JRCGP) and one more general journal (the *British Medical Journal*). I enjoy reading the correspondence columns and these, together with glances through summaries of other articles, hopefully provide a reasonable spectrum of information. For breadth, I ought to read a news-sheet and clinical postgraduate journal, but rarely find time. I find *Prescribers Journal* and the *Drug and Therapeutics Bulletin* good value and only look at advertising material in the journals I referred to above.

In Summary

General day-to-day reading should aim for breadth of cover; depth of cover is best achieved by a specific programme of review. A good up-to-date working knowledge of a field being explored for study can be achieved from a recent paper and its references and working backwards. Review papers, identification of related key issues and of key authors all help. Reference lists and abstracting services can help too but cannot guarantee completeness and are no substitute for personal reading.

Read to confirm that an idea is sensible, read to check that either it is new or there is a reasonable case for repeating previous similar work, read to recognise ways of improving the idea you have and read to learn the weaknesses and strengths of other techniques.

Remember that although it is possible that too much reading may dampen your ability to produce useful original research ideas, too little insults your readers and supporters and wastes your own potential for contributing to the advancement of your subject.

References

Dunlop, D.M., Henderson, T.L. & Inch, R.S., 'A Survey of 17301 Prescriptions on Form EC10', *British Medical Journal*, 1 (1952), pp.292-5.

Elliot, A.E. & Stevenson, J.S.K., 'Geriatric Care in General Practice', *Journal of the Royal College of General Practitioners*, 23 (1973), pp.615-25.

Green, R.H., 'General Practitioners and Open-access Pathology Services', *Journal of the Royal College of General Practitioners*, 23 (1973), pp.316-25.

Lees, D.S. & Cooper, M.H., 'The Work of the General Practitioner', *Journal of the Royal College of General Practitioners*, 6 (1963), pp.408-35.

Louden, I.S.L., 'The General Practitioner and the Hospital', *Trends in General Practice* (Royal College of General Practitioners, London, 1977), pp.83-110.

Reedy, B.L.E.C., 'The Health Team', *Trends in General Practice* (Royal College of General Practitioners, London, 1977), pp.111-41.

Taylor, R.J., 'General Practice Prescribing', *Journal of the Royal College of General Practitioners*, 27 (1977), pp.79-82.

5 THE HYPOTHESIS

Having asked a question, however tentatively, having thought about what the answer might be and how this could be confirmed or the problem explored further, having discussed and read around the theme, it is time to decide the exact aims of the proposed research and to commit these to paper. Without clear aims it is difficult to define appropriate research methods with any confidence and unsatisfactory results will almost inevitably follow. The precise way in which these aims will be stated will necessarily represent the end point of several months of thinking; rushed research is rarely worthwhile and undue haste should be carefully guarded against particularly by those who are relatively inexperienced. During this incubation period the first two criteria of a good research question – interest and importance – will have been well tested. The third criterion of whether or not the question posed is soluble may yet be unanswerable. Further thought on details of design as discussed in the next chapter may suggest either that only a portion of the original question should be tackled or that by reframing the question, more realistic aims can be defined. Whatever the problems this stage of the sequence should always be completed satisfactorily before committing oneself to firm design proposals.

The title of this chapter uses the term 'hypothesis' rather than the more traditional terms 'aims' or 'objectives' to promote the concept that, when possible, research should have as its purpose the answering of specific questions rather than the mere collection of information about a topic. The Shorter Oxford Dictionary defines a hypothesis as: '. . .a supposition in general; something assumed to be true without proof'. Or alternatively as: '. . .a provisional supposition which accounts for known facts and serves as a starting point for further investigation by which it may be proved or disproved'.

A hypothesis may be one in which the research worker believes strongly or may be as weak as a hunch or a feeling; but it will incorporate a degree of commitment to A being true, or B being the cause or explanation of C, or D being a better treatment than E. It is, as Medawar has suggested, 'an informed guess' or 'an imaginative conjecture'. With a hypothesis stated, the subsequent research then centres round proving or disproving the proposition. The discipline of research comes to be seen as necessary and challenging rather than fussy and tedious.

Despite my advocacy of the hypothesis as against the simpler statement of aims, I have to admit that relatively few published papers state a hypothesis. (What I also know is that many of the papers which fail to achieve publication do not even include a clear statement of aims!) Quotation of a number of statements of research aims from successful projects helps to show the range of complexity compatible with success. Waters *et al.* (1976) wrote:

> Comaroff *et al.* reported that 66 per cent of doctors believe that between 1 per cent and 5 per cent of their prescriptions are not dispensed while 20 per cent estimated that all prescriptions they write are dispensed.
>
> This paper reports on the numbers of FP10s and items issued by a general practitioner and his trainee during 1974 and the numbers that were not subsequently dispensed.

The question is 'How many prescriptions are not dispensed?' Reading has shown what doctors *think* is the answer to the question and the research idea is to count how many prescriptions are issued but not apparently dispensed during one year. The implied aim is to convert impressions into numbers in the setting of the authors' practice. It is a good example of simple but sensible research.

> There is no information at present about the proportion of 'out-of-hours' calls being handled by patients' own general practitioners, by their doctors' partners, by doctors in an off-duty rota, or by deputising service doctors. Until we have this information we are in no position to measure the real impact deputising services are making.

Crowe, Hurwood & Taylor (1976) used this quotation from a paper by Williams *et al.* (1973) as the starting point for their descriptive study of a year's out-of-hours calls in their own practice. This demonstrates the usefulness of published work as a source of research questions and again this question is simple enough to suggest a straightforward exercise in documentation of facts.

A clear but more complex statement of aims by Buchan & Richardson (1973) introduced their ambitious and successful 'Time Study of Consultations in General Practice'. They stated:

> The broad aims of the research were, first to measure in units of time all that visibly happens between doctor and patient, and second, to examine the association between certain variables and the duration of both consultation time and its subdivisions. In more specific terms, the aims were:
> 1. To compose a classification of general practitioner activities within direct consultations.
> 2. To devise an appropriate time study technique to measure these activities.
> 3. To examine the effect on length and content of consultations
>   (a) of patient's illness, age, social class
>   (b) of doctor's age, practice location, type and list of size.
> 4. To measure learning effects in a group of trainee assistants.

This clear identification of four discrete aims was later correlated with four separate research exercises; these combined to form the basis of a two-year research fellowship, the results of which were reported as a single Scottish Health Service Study Report.

Watson, Nichols & Robshaw (1975) also deserve commendation for the equally clear statement of aims they used to introduce another relatively complex descriptive study, this time in the field of measles vaccination.

> The aims of this investigation were:
> 1. To study the persistence of haemagglutination inhibiting (HAI) antibody elicited by various types and doses of measles vaccines.
> 2. To seek further evidence of natural boosting by 'wild' measles.
> 3. To study antibody responses after revaccination with a live 'further attenuated' measles vaccine.
> 4. To attempt to correlate antibody responses after revaccination with the type and dose of the primary immunising vaccine, the interval since primary vaccination, and the antibody titre immediately before revaccination.

Some workers come close to proposing a hypothesis when stating their aims but in the end draw back from committing themselves to a particular point of view. Mather *et al.* (1976) in their classic comparison of home and hospital care for patients with myocardial infarction wrote:

> according to some authorities, the mortality of the latter group (home treated) appears to be similar to or lower than that of patients

> treated in hospital. As selection of patients might account for these findings, we planned a randomised controlled trial to compare the fate of patients treated in hospitals. . .with that of patients treated at home.

The fact that published papers frequently state aims and seldom state hypotheses does not necessarily mean that a hypothesis did not exist when the research was initiated. Two papers on the use of cottage hospital beds by general practitioners demonstrate this point. Berkeley stated his aims in two consecutive papers as follows:

> The aim of this study was to determine a rational basis for the provision of general practitioner beds in rural areas (1976a).

> The purpose of this study was to compare the use made of hospital beds in north-east Scotland during a period of one year by a population with access to cottage and general hospital beds, and by a matched population with access only to general medical hospital beds (1976b).

But, in his thesis for the degree of MD (1975) he stated a detailed hypothesis which can be seen to represent the research idea and research question behind the more restricted studies just quoted. The full hypothesis was as follows:

1. In an area without cottage hospital facilities the general practitioner has the option of admitting patients to the central hospital, or treating them at home.
2. In an area with a cottage hospital the general practitioner has the additional option of admitting to the cottage hospital.
3. If the overall in-patient referral rates are the same in the two areas, it is postulated that the patients admitted to the cottage hospital represent a screening off from the central hospital. Secondly, it is postulated that this group of patients are the equivalent of a similar group of patients from the area without cottage hospital facilities, who may be unnecessarily occupying specialised central hospital beds.
4. If the overall in-patient referral rates are higher in the area with cottage hospital facilities, it is further postulated that the excess of patients admitted represent a group of patients who, in the area without such facilities, are receiving extra-hospital care which may not meet their needs.

There *are* examples of hypotheses being quoted in published general practice research literature and two of these illustrate how such statements focus the direction in which the subsequent research will require to be developed.

Hoping to study the effect of 'Night Medication in Rheumatoid Arthritis', Bayley & Haslock (1976) state:

> it has been our practice for some years to give diazepam 10 mg at night under the clinical impression that as well as inducing sleep, the skeletal muscle relaxant property was of value in alleviating morning stiffness.

This study was designed to test this hypothesis and to compare the efficacy of diazepam and indomethacin.

And Taylor *et al.* (1975) prefaced their study of laboratory use by general practitioners with this introduction:

> We have tested the hypothesis that high users of the bacteriology services use some of the investigations often but others rarely. Excessive concentration on the concept that high or low use of investigation is a characteristic of individual doctors or groups of doctors may distract attention from the relevance of many of the investigations to general practice.

This chapter describes one of the relatively few 'mandatory' phases of the research process. At this point, ideas have to be converted to some form of statement of aims so that subsequent plans may be designed to achieve a specific result. The proposal of a hypothesis is a particularly committed way of stating aims, and defining one may seem difficult for those with less experience of research. It is true that before a hypothesis can be proposed some extra thinking is needed about what the research can and should be trying to achieve. But in the end, the statement of a hypothesis will make it easier to design a good and sound project and also more likely that the research will *answer* part of a question, instead of only providing the starting point for further studies.

References

Bayley, T.R.L. & Haslock, I., 'Night Medication in Rheumatoid Arthritis', *Journal of the Royal College of General Practitioners*, 26 (1976), pp.591-4.

Berkeley, J.S., 'The Provision of Cottage Hospital Beds', *Journal of the Royal College of General Practitioners*, 26 (1976a), pp.250-4.

Berkeley, J.S., 'Reasons for Referral to Hospital', *Journal of the Royal College of General Practitioners*, 26 (1976b), pp.293-6.

Berkeley, J.S., 'The Role of the Cottage Hospital', unpublished MD thesis, University of Edinburgh, 1975.

Buchan, I.C. & Richardson, I.M., 'Time Study of Consultations in General Practice', *Scottish Health Service Studies*, no.27 (Scottish Home and Health Department, 1973).

Crowe, M.G.F., Hurwood, D.S. & Taylor, R.W., 'Out-of-hours Calls in a Leicestershire Practice', *British Medical Journal*, 1 (1976), pp.1582-4.

Mather, H.G., Morgan, D.C., Pearson, N.G., Read, K.L.Q., Shaw, D.B., Steed, G.R., Thorne, M.G., Lawrence, C.J., Riley, I.S., 'Myocardial Infarction: A Comparison between Home and Hospital Care for Patients', *British Medical Journal*, 1 (1976), pp.925-9.

Taylor, R.J., Howie, J.G.R., Brodie, J. & Porter, I.A., 'Use of Bacteriological Investigations by General Practitioners', *British Medical Journal*, 3 (1975), pp.635-6.

Waters, W.H.R., Gould, N.V. & Lunn, J.E., 'Undispensed Prescriptions in a Mining General Practice', *British Medical Journal*, 1 (1976), pp.1062-3.

Watson, G.I., Nichols, J.A. & Robshaw, J.R.M., 'Revaccination Against Measles', *Journal of the Royal College of General Practitioners*, 25 (1975), pp.863-73.

Williams, B.T., Dixon, R.A. & Knowelden, J., 'BMA Deputizing Service in Sheffield 1970', *British Medical Journal*, 1 (1973), pp.593-9.

6 SIX IDEAS

This chapter introduces six research projects covering a spread of interests, methods and complexity, and examples of unsuccessful as well as successful research. The examples include research done wholly within the setting of full-time service work as well as that supported by more elaborate technical skills. All the examples are drawn from my own experience of research; my aims are to take the reader behind the scenes of the sometimes artificially tidy final research paper or report, to describe some of the problems which can be expected to arise and to show how some at least can be solved.

As I outline the formative stages of each of these six projects, remember that a good question has been described as one which is important to the doctor asking it (for any one of a number of reasons ranging from its effect on his own workload to the establishment of general principles of good practice), one which is interesting and one which is feasible of solution.

Project One: 'Early or Late Antibiotics in a Flu Epidemic?'

Entering practice in 1966 as a principal with little more than a locum's experience of the problems of general practice, I soon found the management of minor respiratory infection to be one of several areas for which I lacked a working policy. Some colleagues apparently prescribed antibiotics to almost all patients seen – even it seemed on request! – while others prescribed antibiotics relatively infrequently. Viral and bacterial illnesses seemed clinically indistinguishable, side effects of treatment were apparently not common, and 'untreated' patients created awkward problems when they failed to get better as fast as they thought proper. Even if colleagues differed on policies held, they all appeared to use 'experience' as the defence of whatever policy they held and I found this not only unhelpful but a source of disillusionment. My research question was whether or not to prescribe antibiotics routinely at first consultations for minor respiratory illnesses. The question seemed important, not only because the problem was common, but also because no one appeared able to present facts in support of the policies they held. Even to be able to show that unsubstantiated 'experience' did not have to be accepted as the best attainable basis for determining clinical practice seemed a good reason for designing an investigation.

Little happened during the next twelve months. My clinical uncertainty persisted, but acceptance of the *status quo* became easier and began to seem preferable to the alternative of initiating research. Then in January 1968 a *Lancet* editorial on the management of the common cold wrote: 'Until controlled trials in matched populations of sufficient size have demonstrated a clear advantage of antibiotic therapy over placebo under double-blind conditions, the early common cold should have no more than symptomatic treatment.' Within weeks the *Lancet's* correspondence columns carried a letter from Dr Stanley Banks, a retired chest physician, describing work of his own in support of the use of early antibiotic treatment of minor respiratory illness. My growing belief in the need for a clinical trial of early antibiotic use was confirmed; an apparently appropriate research idea had been suggested (by the *Lancet*) and shown to be feasible (by Banks). Banks believed that common colds should be treated within hours of the onset of symptoms: the *Lancet* believed there was insufficient evidence to support such a practice. I hoped to design a study which would choose between the two points of view.

During the summer of 1968 I gained the support of a colleague in a neighbouring practice (Dr G.A. Clark) and we agreed to explore the possibilities of mounting a clinical trial in patients who had – or thought they had – influenza. By autumn 1968 it was clear that the only commercially realistic way to have antibiotics (we had thought of oxytetracycline) and placebos produced was through a pharmaceutical company. A local chemist suggested a company and shortly afterwards I discussed the idea with their local Hospital Manager. By December 1968 we had met one of the company's Medical Advisers, discussed the concept of the study and agreed to draw up proposals for a study. We excused ourselves from reviewing the literature on the grounds that the *Lancet* would have referred to any necessary papers and that Banks' own work provided a quotable paper for balance against the *Lancet* view. The company assured us that they would, in any case, find any necessary references in their own files. Even if our reasoning was naive and in short wrong, our conclusions were probably correct! Before the study could be discussed further, the 1968-9 influenza epidemic emphasised the need for the proposed study, reminded us of the routine practice workload which would co-exist while such a study lasted, and produced a wonderfully useful reference from a ship's surgeon recently involved in managing such an epidemic (Apthorp, 1969). Writing in the *British Medical Journal*, he defined the general practitioner's dilemma (and restated our question) concisely: whether during epidemics of minor respiratory illness, a general practitioner should be an early or a late tetracycline prescriber.

Our question and idea were both clear. Had we precise aims or a hypothesis? In the first protocol submitted to the company we stated, 'We believe that a reasonable policy might be to treat all patients with coryza with a six-day course of a tetracycline derivative starting on the third day of the illness if signs or symptoms of lower respiratory disease are present – usually cough with or without sputum.'

This was the nearest we came to defining aims at any stage and the eventual paper reporting on this work claimed in very general terms to 'describe a trial designed to provide some of the evidence lacking on these points (benefits and risks of antibiotic against no-antibiotic in patients with flu-like illnesses)'. Without a hypothesis to test, we were not forced to decide in advance what difference between the groups would be taken as clinically significant and ended with a study able only to describe the natural history of influenzal illnesses in antibiotic and placebo takers. Identification of significant differences between the groups – the true aim of the study – could become a possibility only if enough patients were, by chance, studied and we were to be grateful for the 1969-70 influenza epidemic which rescued us from a fundamental weakness in our preliminary thinking about this project. Without the considerable quantity of material this epidemic produced, we could have ended with an inconclusive and unsatisfactory study.

For this investigation two years elapsed between asking the question and starting to design the project in detail. A further year was to pass before collection of results began. We asked a good question and had a good idea; but we should have reviewed the literature more adequately and we should have defined more precise aims or preferably have stated a hypothesis. (The project designed for this investigation is outlined on page 101.)

Project Two: 'Do "Diagnoses" Determine or Justify Management Decisions?'

Traditional teaching has always stressed the importance of making a diagnosis as an intermediate stage between taking a history (in the broad sense including examination and investigation) and deciding management. My observations of hospital clinicians at work, both when I was an undergraduate and as a postgraduate, made me sceptical of the universal application of this principle and fairly certain that many acute decisions were taken largely on emotional or pragmatic grounds, later justified by forcing 'evidence' into awkwardly unwelcoming diagnostic pigeon-holes. Early in my own experience of general practice, I realised that this was a common pattern in my own making of clinical decisions. Within seconds of seeing an unwell-looking coughing baby I would have decided to prescribe an antibiotic; the next three minutes were spent finding evidence to support an already made decision. Slight pinkness of an ear-drum readily became inflammation, redness of a throat inflammation as against injection, and so on. Referrals to hospital, decisions to revisit, the content of certificates were all capable of being justified by emphasising selected aspects of history taking and examination and my second research question became 'How central is the making of a traditional "diagnosis" to general practice decisions on management?' The question seemed important because discussion of clinical problems inevitably centred around diagnostic terms although the criteria for using them were rarely discussed. 'All patients with tracheitis require an antibiotic' – but what is tracheitis? 'All patients with mesenteric adenitis should be in hospital' – but what is mesenteric adenitis? 'All patients with depression should be on anti-depressant' – but what is depression? Once again it seemed that when doctors were challenged on their widely different use of diagnostic terms they resorted to using their 'experience' as their defence. It seemed likely to me that 'experience' was a worthwhile concept and that general practitioners probably had much more in common in what they did than in the way they explained what they did. It was my belief that the uncritical use of often unsuitable diagnostic terms was retarding the establishment of the clinical identity of the discipline and its practitioners.

The analysis of clinical information gathered during the north-east Scotland workload study had shown widely variable use, both of diagnostic labels and of antibiotics in the management of respiratory illnesses (Howie *et al.*, 1971). My research idea was to collect further information on the signs and symptoms of respiratory illness which doctors thought influenced them at individual consultations, note the diagnoses they recorded and the treatment they prescribed and then make simple correlations. My hypothesis was that there would be a better correlation between *clinical information collected* and *treatment given*, than between either *clinical information collected* and *diagnosis made*, or *diagnosis made* and *treatment given.* My hope was to be able to show that this hypothesis was right in the setting of new consultations for respiratory illness; I did not wish to suggest that it necessarily applied to all illnesses or all consultations. But I believed that until the profession had recognised its reality, both teaching and clinical practice would inevitably be founded on an unsatisfactory basis. I also believed that the poor esteem in which general practice was often held by specialist colleagues stemmed from our inability to present the unique difficulties and challenges of our own job in terms of our own choosing.

I reviewed the literature from British general practice fairly thoroughly and found little helpful to this idea. Had I read the work of Feinstein (1967) at this stage, the appropriateness of my hypothesis would have been confirmed, but I might have been dissuaded from testing it because of its overlap with his earlier researches in the setting of American hospital medicine. The question was one which seemed of real importance to me; the idea seemed simple and the clear wording of the hypothesis suggested – correctly – that the design of the study would be relatively straightforward. (The design used is described on page 108.)

Project Three: 'Co-trimoxazole and Streptococcal Tonsillitis'

This, the third of my six projects, was the least satisfactory. In July 1974 I was approached by a pharmaceutical company anxious to set up a study of the effectiveness of co-trimoxazole in treating streptococcal throat infections. The company had evidence that the drug was effective against the organism in the laboratory and wished to be able to market the drug as a reserve treatment for patients unable to receive penicillin because of allergy. Because previous clinical trials using standard dosage of co-trimoxazole had shown incomplete eradication of the streptococcus, the proposal was to increase the drug dosage from the average to the maximum recommended dose (three tablets twice daily against two tablets twice daily). On the surface this would appear a straightforward project; the question was simple (does a given dose of the test drug have comparable efficiency with penicillin against the organism concerned?) and the idea of a clinical trial seemed feasible. It was further agreed that we use the study as an opportunity to measure the efficiency of seven-day courses of penicillin. (Wannamaker had shown in 1953 that five-day courses were ineffective in eradicating streptococci and most doctors accept that ten-day courses are rarely completed.) Although no hypothesis was stated the principal aim of the study was defined clearly as 'to compare the efficacy of high dose co-trimoxazole and oral penicillin V in the treatment of Group A beta-haemolytic streptococcal throat infections'.

Looking at this with hindsight, the main reasons for its eventual difficulties (described in Chapters 10 and 13) were that the questions asked did not adequately meet the criteria of interest and importance. Although the research was interesting and important to the company concerned because it might provide evidence to support a new area of promotion, it was of interest and importance to me more as an opportunity to examine the feasibility of organising good-quality clinical trials in local teaching practices (although I accepted that the trial was a justifiable and ethically sound clinical exercise). But the critical weakness was that the study proved of insufficient interest or importance to the local general practitioners who agreed to collect patients. The lesson from this is now indelibly written on my mind. Do not undertake research unless you both believe in its importance and feel that the subject of study is one in which you have a genuine interest. A neutral position on either count soon becomes a negative one and that spells almost certain failure. (The next stage in the development of this project is described on page 112.)

Project Four: 'The Prevention of Adverse Drug Reactions'

This project was probably the simplest of the six. In 1974 I was involved, along with Dr Denis Durno and a colleague in the local University Department of Therapeutics (Dr J.C. Petrie), in a study of general practitioners' knowledge of the risks of drug interactions. One of the findings of possible clinical importance was the low proportion of general practitioners aware of the risks of interaction between warfarin and barbiturates, although this particular interaction is one of those most likely to have serious clinical implications. After this study, two warning labels were prepared, one for attachment to the record envelope of patients at risk (Figure 6.1) and the other for tagging, either to a drug record held inside the wallet, or to the continuation notes if preferred (Figure 6.2).

The question was simple: would the use of warning labels of this kind reduce the risk of vulnerable patients receiving potentially dangerous combinations of drugs? We were familiar with the literature on communication of drug information between hospital and general practitioner and knew of no previous attempt to assess the value of such a method. The idea which developed involved identifying all patients on anticoagulants in our unusually well-defined local hospital area and dividing them into two groups. The doctors of patients in one group would be sent the warning labels, the more detailed one being attached to a 'drug card' as shown in Figure 6.3.

Figure 6.1: Warning Label for Record Envelope

WARNING

ANTICOAGULANT INTERACTIONS

Figure 6.2: Warning Label for Continuation Notes or Drug Card

ANTICOAGULANT INTERACTIONS

Barbiturates, sedatives (not nitrazepam), alcohol, sulphonamides, phenylbutazone, clofibrate, nalidixic acid, mefenamic acid, indomethacin, phenytoin, aspirin ($>$2g/day), sulphonylureas, griseofulvin, quinidine, vitamin C, oral contraceptives, laxatives, ethacrynic acid, ? broad spectrum antibiotics.

The doctors of patients in the second group would receive only the 'drug card' as control, but neither label. After six months the drugs prescribed to the two groups of patients would be compared. The study was described as an 'evaluation of a warning system designed to increase the awareness of doctors of potential adverse drug interactions' and the hypothesis was that use of the system would reduce the number of potentially interacting drugs prescribed to patients at risk. It is worth stressing the simplicity of the question asked and the hypothesis put under test. It was tempting to postulate that increased awareness and reduced prescription of at-risk drugs would improve quality of care, but

Surname | First Names

Address

Date	DRUG	Strength of tablet etc.	Quantity Prescribed

ANTICOAGULANT INTERACTIONS

Barbiturates, sedatives (not nitrazepam), alcohol, sulphonamides, phenylbutazone, clofibrate, nalidixic acid, mefenamic acid, indomethacin, phenytoin, aspirin ($>$2g/day), sulphonylureas, griseofulvin, quinidine, vitamin C, oral contraceptives, laxatives, ethacrynic acid, ? broad spectrum antibiotics.

to test this would have required the collection of accurate information on drugs taken as well as drugs prescribed. Estimation of serial prothrombin times from up to 400 mobile patients distributed over an area of some 3,000 square miles would have been required. We recognised practical difficulties in achieving this level of follow-up and opted for the simple and probably feasible study in preference to the more complex study with the much lower chance of being successfully concluded. (Further details of the planning of the study are discussed on page 115.)

Project Five: 'Can Clinical Judgement be Analysed?'

After spending a number of years attempting to demonstrate that the clinical decisions of general practice were capable of analysis, I had concluded that right (and thus wrong) approaches to the clinical management of common problems could be defined, practised and taught. I now found myself anxious to establish the scientific respectability of the 'art' of the general practitioner – best summarised as his ability to make judgements on clinical matters which balance illness factors and patient factors in an informed and appropriate way. Richardson (1975) had defined the criteria of an independent clinical discipline as the responsibility for a distinctive cross-section of illness, the possession of special skills and the application of a characteristic philosophy. The independent scope and nature of general practice work has not been in doubt for many years and the clinical skill of differentiating the component parts of non-specific illness quickly, and without the routine use of investigation, is surely particular to general practice. My belief was that for general practice to be assured of academic acceptability equal to that of established hospital disciplines, it was still necessary to quantify the particular philosophy which marked general practice medicine as different from, though complementary to, hospital medicine. This difference in philosophy is, I believe, the relative (not absolute) importance which general practitioners properly accord to patient as against illness factors in making their clinical judgements – I have amplified on this elsewhere (Howie, 1978). My research question was, 'Can I demonstrate how "patient" factors influence the clinical decisions taken by general practitioners?'

Without doubt this was a most difficult question to answer by research. My reading of Feinstein's *Clinical Judgement* (1967) encouraged me to persist in trying to find an answer to my question, and some success with the use of simulated consultations in earlier research (Howie, 1974) encouraged the development of an idea. The idea required presentation of standard physical (illness) information together with variable non-physical (patient) information to a number of general practitioners and noting the decisions on management they claimed they would take. If change of 'patient' information could be shown to significantly alter actions normally regarded in hospital as being determined wholly on 'illness' criteria, I should have strong circumstantial evidence in support of my belief. I had to show that using simulated material was valid, and identifying a clinical topic where decisions to use physical treatment might be influenced by non-physical factors. Once again the antibiotic appeared the easiest treatment to investigate and sore throat the ideal clinical topic. Verbal diagnostic and descriptive statements regarding 'pharyngitis' and 'tonsillitis', 'inflammation' and 'injection' seemed poor starting points for clinical simulations which had to be accepted as realistic, and I decided to explore the use of photography and reproduction as the means of producing standard clinical material. The eventual success of the venture owed much to the enthusiasm and devotion of the professional medical illustrators (Richard Morton and Ted Smith) who agreed willingly to support this apparently untried research approach.

In this project the hypothesis 'that awareness of non-physical features in a consultation for physical illness (in this case the symptom of sore throat with the sign of localised redness) may influence in a measurable way the doctor's decision to prescribe a physical remedy (in this case an antibiotic)' was coupled with a subsidiary or fail-safe aim, namely an attempt to demonstrate 'the feasibility of designing studies capable of examining the components of clinical judgement in general practice'.

Like many projects the process of question-idea-hypothesis was a progressively evolving one with the eventual hypothesis being proposed only after much discussion, general rather than particular reading, and the realisation that a practical idea was available. From the time of first thinking about the possibility of the project to starting to design it, the study took some three to four years. Amazingly, from starting the design to publication of the results took less than ten months. Time spent in adequate thinking about research is always repaid in the later stages of the work – usually in terms of time saved and almost always in terms of the quality of the results obtained. (The methods used to develop this research interest are described on page 117.)

Project Six: 'Prescribing to Save Work'

One of the most common and honest reasons given for prescribing antibiotics for minor respiratory illnesses is the belief that patients want them and will make extra calls (particularly at night) if these drugs are not prescribed. The alternative point of view is that prescribing an antibiotic for one illness conditions the patient to consult again when next complaining of the same illness, and that symptomatic treatment of the first illness might encourage the patient to self-treat when ill subsequently. There are, of course, caveats to be expressed on the consequences of both policies but no evidence is available to allow an informed choice to be made between these different policies, either on operational or clinical grounds.

The problems faced either by a trainee working in a practice where doctors differ in broad prescribing strategy from each other or by a trainee wishing to prescribe differently from existing practice policy, are ones which many doctors will now have experienced. This project describes an attempt which I made with a general practice trainee (Dr Katherine Hutchison) to answer the question 'Does a doctor with a lower prescribing policy (for antibiotics in respiratory illness) than other doctors in a practice create extra work for his partners?' Being a project intended to assist a trainee in training it was desirable that the results should become available during the training year and the fieldwork had to be undertaken and completed quickly. The question was asked in January 1976 and had to be answered by June 1976. Even if this is not the ideal time setting for research, much can be achieved in a short time and much learned about the difficulties of collecting good-quality information and interpreting 'facts'.

The research idea was to use existing practice records to assess how often patients seen by the various doctors in the practice made further consultations for respiratory illness within two weeks of an apparently new consultation and

(a) received an antibiotic when one had not been prescribed initially, or
(b) received a change of antibiotic after an antibiotic had been prescribed initially.

The limitations of the idea were recognised and we knew that the conclusions might be personal to the doctors rather than generally applicable. Without any idea of what would be found and how suitable the information from the routine records would prove to be, no hypothesis was stated. The aims were no more than to explore whether the idea described would be capable of helping answer the question; it was hoped that if the study did prove successful it might be used as a pilot study leading to the statement of a specific hypothesis for further study. Although the study was a modest one, a high level of interest in its outcome was maintained during the short time it lasted. Simple research tends to generate a momentum of its own and often leads to further research. Over-ambitious research kills interest and curiosity with alarming finality. (The further planning of this study is outlined on page 124.)

These six projects can be seen separately as representing something of the variety of ways in which an individual doctor can develop a research interest of his own; or they may be viewed together as showing how diverse one person's research interest can become as each project appears to pose more questions than it answers. I hope that the overall effect of this chapter will have been to show that research is not an ivory-tower activity undertaken to produce 'publications', but an activity making a creative contribution to the understanding, teaching and practice of medicine generally. It is idle to think that general practice can develop – or indeed hold its ground – without a research contribution; it is, however, important that that contribution should be a sound one. The next section discusses the principles of research design in some detail and in Chapter 10 I will discuss the application of these principles to the projects I have introduced in this chapter.

References

Apthorp, B.D., 'Hong Kong Influenza', *British Medical Journal*, 1 (1969), p.49.
Banks, H.S., 'Antibiotics and the Common Cold', *Lancet*, 1 (1968), pp.425-6.
Feinstein, A.R., *Clinical Judgement* (Williams & Wilkins, Baltimore, 1967).
Howie, J.G.R., 'Further Observations on Diagnosis and Management of General Practice Respiratory Illness Using Simulated Patient Consultations', *British Medical Journal*, 2 (1974), pp.540-3.
Howie, J.G.R., 'The Art and the Epidemiologist', *Journal of the Royal College of General Practitioners*, 28 (1978), pp.71-7.
Howie, J.G.R., Richardson, I.M., Gill, G. & Durno, D., 'Respiratory Illness and Antibiotic Use in General Practice', *Journal of the Royal College of General Practitioners*, 21 (1971), pp.657-63.
Lancet, leading article, 'Antibiotics and the Common Cold', 1 (1968), p.240.
Petrie, J.C., Howie, J.G.R. & Durno, D., 'Awareness and Experience of General Practitioners of Selected Drug Interactions', *British Medical Journal*, 2 (1974), pp.262-4.

Richardson, I.M., 'The Value of a University Department of General Practice', *British Medical Journal*, 4 (1975), pp.740-2.
Wannamaker, L.W. *et al.*, 'The Effect of Penicillin Prophylaxis on Streptococcal Disease Rates and the Carrier State', *New England Journal of Medicine*, 249 (1953), pp.1-7.

PART TWO

DOING RESEARCH

7 DESIGNING STUDIES

Designing a research project is like composing a recipe for cooking. The designer wants to lay out a stage-by-stage description of the ingredients required and the way they are to be used. Recipes for simple dishes are usually simple; those for cordon bleu cooking more complex. Good recipes state precise weights and suggest exact oven temperatures; those describing teacupsful and 'hot' ovens produce uncertain results. So it is for research; simple projects can be carried out using very simple plans whereas projects aiming to answer complex problems will usually need more elaborate planning. Attention to detail is repaid when the time comes to analyse results.

A chapter on research design could be a long one. An extensive literature on the subject already exists and specialist books (such as Witts' on surveys and clinical trials, and Bennett & Ritchie's on the use of questionnaires in medicine) have been written on single aspects of research design. My purpose is to identify the more important issues which have to be settled before collection of results can begin and to comment on their application to research in general practice.

Almost any research involves the collection of information for numerical analysis, normally in some form of 'rate' – for example, consultations per hour, prescriptions issued per patient per year. The figure on the top line is the *numerator* and refers to the event or phenomenon being studied (consultations or prescriptions in these examples). The lower figure is the *denominator* and refers to the population (or sample of the population) in which the event/phenomenon was studied (hours or patients and years in these examples). The first two parts of this chapter comment on the choosing of the numerator and denominator. Later parts discuss some of the methods available for collecting research information, and give guidance on selecting the size and scope of different kinds of studies. The final part of the chapter examines some of the ethical issues which are raised by research in general practice.

The Numerator

The terms 'event' and 'phenomenon' are frequently used to indicate the subject which will form the numerator when the results of the study come to be analysed. The ideal event is one which is:

easily defined;
easily recognised when it *is* present;
not identified when it *is not* present; and
occurs commonly enough, or is significant enough for interest in and awareness of its occurrence to be maintained.

Some events clearly fulfil these criteria. Death is one; so is the writing of a prescription, or the carrying out of a home visit, or the measuring of a blood pressure or the taking of a cervical smear. These items are easily recognised and not likely to be thought present in error. They are, in other words, objective terms. Although some terms may be so unambiguous as to require no further description, other apparently objective terms may require additional definitions when being used for research purposes. One example of how confusion may arise is in the use of the term 'night call'. Many doctors would regard a night call as one received after the doctor has gone to bed; others might feel that any call qualifying for extra payment should be included and define the night call as one between 11.00 pm and 7.00 am. Again, others might regard any call after 6.00 pm as a night call, although calls between 6.00 pm and 11.00 pm are usually labelled simply late calls. But late calls have been defined in some circumstances as calls received after 11.00 am on a normal working day! The exact definition chosen is a matter for the choice of the individual research planner. What is essential is that the criteria he chooses are clearly defined so that all collaborators include identical material and, later on, those reading the results know what is being described.

When terms have a commonly used meaning, for instance, 'direct consultation', 'complete appointments system', there is merit in keeping to this for a research study. The risk of misinterpreting reported results is reduced and comparison of findings with other published work is often made easier. For the purposes of general practice research, the Royal College of General Practitioners has produced a glossary of terms which may assist in choosing definitions of key items for research studies. This is available as a fifteen-page document, published as supplement three to volume 23 (1973) of the JRCGP. It is well worth reading at this stage of designing a research project.

Having so far commented almost entirely on the more easily defined administrative or operational terms which may be used, I want to urge caution on the use of diagnostic labels as numerator information. Doctors vary greatly in the way they respond to symptoms presented by their patients. Some carry out more physical examination than others; some investigate and refer more than others. Labels of obesity in patients who have not been weighed, of bronchitis in patients whose chests have not been examined, of urinary infection in patients from whom no specimens have been cultured, or of migraine in patients whose self-diagnoses are accepted without question, clearly provide an unsafe basis for research work. And these are only a few examples of many which could be used to illustrate the objectivity of diagnostic labels as used in day-to-day practice. In routine clinical discussions within a practice their meaning to the doctors using them may become familiar and satisfactory (for insurance certification and other such purposes they are again useful and satisfactory), but for research they are both inadequate and often frankly misleading. It is highly desirable that any general practice research project of a clinical nature defines in as exact terms as possible the precise conditions to be met for any diagnostic term which is to be used in the study.

There are two further points to be covered at this stage. First, it may be necessary to define not only the end-point of an event, but also the process by which it was reached. A negative result from a throat swab examined two hours after being taken has a quite different significance from a similar result from a swab not plated until 48 hours after it was taken; and a fourth phase diastolic blood pressure recorded in an obese sitting patient being seen for the first time is not comparable with a fifth phase reading in a thin recumbent patient who attends for this examination on a regular basis. Thus, criteria for the definition of key events should include sufficient detail to prevent inaccuracies from variations in the methods used to make the observations. Second, the difference between the *incidence* and the *prevalence* of events has to be understood. Incidence is the number of new occurrences of an event in a defined population during a stated period of observation, whereas the prevalence of an event includes all events (say illnesses) beginning during the period and either ending during the period or lasting beyond it; all those starting before, but ending during the period; and all those starting before and persisting after the period. These points are illustrated in Figure 7.1; only illnesses A and B count in a study of incidence; all four would be included in a study of prevalence. Prevalence may be divided into period prevalence (where prevalence over an interval of time is noted) and point prevalence (where the prevalence at one set moment is noted).

Figure 7.1: Incidence and Prevalence

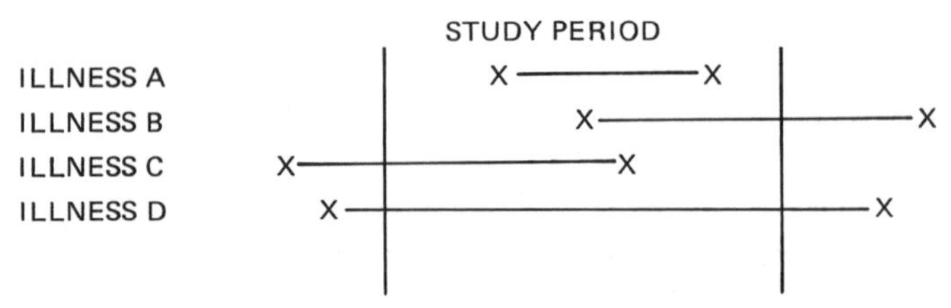

The Denominator

Having decided what is to be studied and how it is to be defined it is necessary to decide where to look for this information. Smoking habits of *teenage males*; treatment of *patients with acne*; the length of consultations for *patients with headache* – in these examples the denominator is shown in italics. Just as with information required for the numerator, the definition of the denominator should be carefully and clearly stated. 'Teenage males' are readily recognisable; 'patients with acne' or 'patients with headache' may be less so.

The main issue to decide is whether to study a population or a sample from a population. A population implies a complete group of people, patients, consultations or whatever is being surveyed. 'Teenage males' would imply all teenage males whereas what is probably intended would be 'teenage males registered with practice X' or some similar variant of a smaller sample population. If the study is to be of patients consulting the doctor rather than persons registered with the doctor, then this must also be stated because of course differences between 'consulting' and 'non-consulting' patients may reflect important differences not only in physical well-being but also in attitudes to, for example, self-treatment or dependence on professional reassurance. Thus, the denominator may be expanded again to become 'teenage males in practice X consulting. . .with respiratory symptoms during November' and so on. If a complete and adequately defined population is chosen for study the results can later be compared more readily with those from other studies involving similar populations. Either all patients who qualify as part of the defined population must be studied or conditions for exclusions must be stated and note made of all who are subsequently left out of the study.

At the same time as the population is being defined, consideration should be given to groups within the population which might later be of interest as sub-populations. Common divisions include age, sex, occupation and social class, marital state, past history of illness; many other qualities could be added and each one selected has to be capable of definition. These additional items which describe a population more fully are often called 'variables' and research design should include plans to note information about major or potentially useful variables. However, the temptation to record every conceivable variable 'on the off-chance' should be resisted. Beyond a certain point complexity of design adversely affects the quality of the data which is collected and reduces the willingness of others to collaborate. On the whole, the simpler the aims of the study, the fewer the variables that have to be noted.

The basic problems of defining a numerator and denominator are thus similar and during the analysis of results what is used as a numerator in one analysis (*'number of teenagers smoking 20 cigarettes per day in practice X'*) may be used as the whole or part of the denominator in a subsequent analysis ('breakdown by social class of *teenagers smoking 20 cigarettes per day in practice X'*).

Samples

A sample is part of a complete population. A properly drawn sample should reflect the attributes of the original population both in nature and in proportion. In populations where biological and behavioural characteristics are present it is always possible that significant but undefined properties of the original population will be missed or over-represented when a sample is taken; such a sample is thus not representative of the population from which it has been drawn and is described as biased. The aim of sampling is to reduce the risk of sampling bias to the minimum. Again, as in the case of a population, the way in which the sample is to be or has been drawn must be stated accurately and completely and the exact description of the original population repeated. When a sample is drawn correctly, the risk of bias which is present in any sampling procedure will be higher in small samples and reduced in large samples.

There are two particular kinds of sampling which should be mentioned at this stage. In a *stratified* sample various groups in the whole population are separated before the sample is drawn and the whole sample then composed from the sub-groups in a predetermined fashion. Out of, for example, 500 members of a church, 300 might be female and 200 male. If a sample of 100 is wanted it might be agreed that equal numbers of each sex should be included. Thus, to obtain 50 females and 50 males, one in six females and one in four males would require to be identified.

The second kind of sample is the *random* sample, in which each member of the population has an equal chance of being chosen in the sample. Random sampling implies a positive decision to use random sampling techniques and not simply the absence of a decision to select from a complete population in a particular way. In strict terms taking every tenth patient is a systematic and not a random sample and would, for example, introduce bias in a study of surgery consultations by over-representing the first booked patient who is more likely than average to be a return booking. However, by randomising the starting point for identification of patient one, a satisfactory compromise would be effected. Although drawing numbers from a hat is a satisfactory sampling technique, random number tablets are included in most books on statistics to aid the collection of truly representative samples.

The risks of haphazard sampling include bias towards a particular number by the sampler (most people show what is called 'digit preference') or use of unbalanced aids – a telephone directory may contain more of particular numbers because of biases introduced by local code prefixes.

In general practice research a number of aids to the drawing of samples have been in use for many years. Each has advantages and disadvantages. The most useful aid is the age-sex register. Using cards, available through the Royal College of General Practitioners (Figure 7.2) or specifically constructed for the purpose, a list of patients registered with a practice is compiled and stored in age order with male and female patients separated. A variety of samples can easily be drawn from such files. The weakness of these indexes lies in the rate at which they become inaccurate if not kept up to date. Old patients tend to be over-represented unless care is taken to remove records of those who have died; newborn children may be under-represented because of their parents' failure to register them. There will be false inclusions of patients who have moved away but not reported this fact and omissions of those who regard themselves as under the care of the practice but have not yet registered.

Disease indexes can be constructed either from routine continuous recording, or from selected recording of morbidity seen by a doctor or a practice, and the E-book system – described in Eimerl & Laidlaw's *A Handbook for Research in General Practice* (1969) – is one way in which this can be done. Indexes of this kind are satisfactory bases for research sampling only so long as clearly defined criteria for inclusion and exclusion of episodes of illness under the various disease headings have (i) been stated and (ii) are known to have been universally and

Figure 7.2: Age-sex Register Card (Royal College of General Practitioners)

A.S.R.2a **COLLEGE OF GENERAL PRACTITIONERS RECORDS and STATISTICS UNIT**

Card	Dr. Code							Surname of Patient			Forename	Date of Birth			Sex	MS	SS
1	2	3	4	5	6	7	8	9	10	11	12	13-14	15-16	17-18	19	20	21

Addresses		E.C.
1.	N.H.S. No.	
	Date (Entry)	22-23 / 24-25 / 26-27
2.		
	Date (Removal)	28-29 / 30-31 / 32-33
3.		
	Reason	34 / 35
Occupation		
	Card to E.C. / /19	

A	B	C	D	E	F	G	H	I	J	K	L	M	N	O	P	Q	R	S	T	U	V	W	X	Y	Z
36	37	38	39	40	41	42	43	44	45	46	47	48	49	50	51	52	53	54	55	56	57	58	59	60	61

consistently applied throughout the period during which the index or register has been compiled. This is rarely the case and I personally have misgivings about research which is based on populations or samples drawn from such sources.

A research worker may find it difficult to decide whether he should study a whole population which is readily available to him or should sample from a larger population which is, however, less accessible. Very different results may be produced.

> Westcott (1977) studied the time taken for 44 'psychoneurotic' consultations and found a mean time of 14 minutes; Buchan & Richardson (1973) studied 124 such consultations and found a mean time of 5.3 minutes.
>
> Westcott studied a population of his own consultations during two weeks in November. Buchan & Richardson sampled six sessions of work during a year from 24 doctors and thus report about an average of five such consultations per doctor. Westcott's study tells more about psychoneurotic consultations generally. (This, of course, begs the question of how a 'psychoneurotic' consultation can be defined objectively!) On the surface the two papers are

> comparable; but closer study shows Westcott's report relates to one trainee year whereas Buchan and Richardson's study covers the work of a selection of principals in practice.
>
> Each study has a contribution to make, but in the contexts of the denominators defined for each separately; the two are complementary but not directly comparable.

It is wise to take advice before a final decision is taken on the denominator to be used, as the direction of the research may be greatly influenced by the choice. Whatever the choice that is made, the population must be defined as exactly as possible and any sampling method used described equally carefully.

Types of Research

A variety of terms are used to describe the different kinds of research which are commonly undertaken in a medical setting. 'Operational research', 'morbidity studies', 'workload studies', 'clinical research' are no more than descriptive terms implying the kind of subjects which they cover. No individual principles of design are applicable to any one, although different emphases will be appropriate to particular projects.

There are, however, two contrasting tactical approaches to research (retrospective and prospective research) and the different strengths and weaknesses of each should be understood before a research plan is agreed. In addition, particular problems arise when attempts are being made to compare (as against describe) methods of clinical management (clinical trials); again anticipation of problems is much to be preferred to attempting, usually unsatisfactorily, late repair of damage due to faulty design.

Retrospective and Prospective Research

The principal difference between retrospective and prospective research is that retrospective research analyses material which is already available and has not been collected with the aims of the specific project in mind, whereas prospective research is designed to collect new information for later analysis.

Retrospective research can relatively easily survey very large quantities of information from many sources. It can conveniently cover greater periods of time than is often feasible in prospective research. Information available is, however, rarely of definable or standard quality and its accuracy may thus be very difficult to judge. In the same vein, it is often difficult to assess the population from which the information was obtained. As a result, what becomes available is likely to be of desirable quantity but uncertain quality; and the information, although often capable of showing associations between factors studied, can rarely comment on the nature of such associations.

Prospective research can be purpose built and allows greater control over the quality of information collected. The main disadvantage usually lies in the smaller amount of material which can be collected during a reasonable period of time and from a workable number of patients or practices. Moreover, the risk of bias on the part of the observer becomes an additional consideration. If a prospective study is well designed, cause and effect relationships may be identifiable, and this, of course, is of particular value when the cause of an illness is being sought or the effectiveness of a treatment is being tested.

In theoretical terms an end-point D may be observed in a retrospective study and items A, B and C found to be associated. It may be suggested that

$$A + B + C \longrightarrow D$$

but it is unlikely that retrospective research will allow comment to be made with any confidence on whether $A + B \longrightarrow D$ or $A + C \longrightarrow D$ or whether A and B react to produce X which then reacts with C to give D, and so on. Particularly in the setting of biological research, it cannot be accurately guaged how often A + B + C will give D as the degree to which A, B, C and D represent all of A, B, C, D or include wrongly identified A, B, C and D will usually be a matter for conjecture rather than certainty. Normally a prospective study will be needed if items A, B and C are to be identified accurately and added together in various orders or watched interacting spontaneously so that their contributions to causing D can be more fully analysed and quantified.

In practical terms, the original association between, for example, cigarette smoking and bronchial cancer followed retrospective study of patients with carcinoma of lung and investigation of records of smoking habits. A prospective study of defined populations then identified improved prognoses for non-smokers and ex-smokers and comes as near to showing cause and effect as is possible (although not proving cause and effect as a further common, but still unidentified link – say genetic – between smokers and cancer sufferers could of course exist). Quite often a retrospective study based on a 'hunch' provides evidence suggesting a prospective analysis of the topic concerned is justifiable.

In the setting of general practice research, the retrospective studies of practice records with which Fry's name has become synonymous have been of major value in outlining the clinical territory of general practice; but such information is not particularly suited to the evaluation of alternative approaches to clinical care. Prospective projects such as Everett's simple study of antibiotic against placebo in management of diarrhoeal illness (1973) are now needed as attempts are made to define quality in patient care.

Clinical Trials

The clinical trial is a particular variety of prospective research in which say treatment A and treatment B are compared in management of disease X. The ideal trial involves random allocation of treatments A and B to one population of patients with disease X. Takers of treatments A and B become samples and the larger the samples, the more likely it is that the samples will be identical in enough important factors to be comparable, 'treatment taken' remaining as the main likely contributor to any difference in outcome which is observed. Random allocation of patients between treatment groups should allow unsuspected biological variables to be distributed equally between the two groups being compared but this is not itself adequate for many purposes. Behavioural influences must also be considered. Not only do doctors want to see the treatments they prescribe as being beneficial, but patients, too, like to feel that the drugs (or other measures) they have been prescribed have been of value. In the ideal clinical trial, neither the doctor giving treatment (or analysing the results) nor the patient receiving it should know which treatment has been used. Such a trial is described as *double-blind.* Where either doctor or patient (but not both) knows the treatment allocated the study is described as *single-blind.* Clearly ethical difficulties have to be considered (see page 86) and the nature of the trial or study may make random allocation to treatments impossible – for example, the oral contraceptive study (RCGP, 1974) where pill-takers and non pill-takers were compared – or double-blind design impractical – say hypnotism compared with liquid nitrogen in treatment of warts. Elaborations of double-blind trials include those where treatments are alternated as a trial progresses (cross-over studies) but such studies are normally initiated from outside rather than within general practice.

When the term 'controlled' is included in the description of a clinical trial this implies that patients receiving the test treatment are to be matched and compared with others receiving another treatment or receiving no treatment. For the reasons already mentioned, when the patients acting as 'controls' are to receive no active treatment, it is preferable that a placebo should be used. A description of the outcome of a single treatment with no controls included is notoriously difficult to interpret, and results from this kind of research are readily open to abuse. Doctors asked to collaborate in clinical trials should be as critical of the research design of such trials as they would be when constructing studies of their own. I, myself, would not normally be willing to participate in a drug trial which was not adequately controlled and experience has taught me that 'adequately controlled' will normally mean that treatment takers and controls are selected on a 'double-blind' basis.

Methods of Collecting Information

Once the details required for the numerator and denominator have been decided and a broad strategy outlined, the methods to be used to collect the information have to be chosen. A variety of techniques are in common use and the value of many of them has been proved by successful application. Other methods are less well established and the need to experiment with new techniques of study is as real in general practice as in any other developing discipline.

Validity and Reliability. An ideal method of collecting research information is one which is valid and reliable. A valid method is one which measures what it sets out to measure; a reliable method is one which produces repeatable results.

The difference between validity and reliability can be illustrated by considering an example: the estimation of haemoglobin by colorimetric tests on a finger-stab blood sample is suitable to this purpose. The estimation provides a *valid* test of the blood's haemoglobin concentration provided that:

haemoglobin concentration in the blood in the finger mirrors haemoglobin concentration elsewhere;
the chemical treatment of the blood before assessing its optical qualities does not destroy relevant components of the blood;
the standard with which the test is compared is known to reflect a given concentration of haemoglobin correctly.

The estimation is *reliable* if:

the haemoglobin concentration in the finger remains constant at,

for example, different temperatures of the body;
the chemical reaction is instant (or its rate is known) and remains stable for the time required;
different observers, or the same observer at different times, will agree over the dilution of the test specimen which is needed before test and control colour intensities are balanced.

Validity and reliability are of course relative concepts and what constitutes an acceptable degree of either has to be considered in the context of a given study; sickness certificates appear to be a valid method for charting the spread of an influenza epidemic from region to region, but cannot be used as a valid method of identifying patients developing true influenza when attempting to assess the effectiveness of a vaccine. Similarly, a method of estimating haemoglobin which is sufficiently reliable to support decisions for or against the need for emergency blood transfusion may not be sufficiently reliable for the exclusion of early megaloblastic anaemia in the elderly.

Direct observation of a doctor consulting will be a reliable method for recording how many patients have been weighed or had their temperatures taken during a period of observation; but if the presence of the observer has changed the doctor's normal habits, this method would not be a valid way of assessing that doctor's normal behaviour. Examination of night-visit claim forms may be a valid way of attempting to identify a group of patients who have received night visits, but it is not a reliable way of identifying all such patients because doctors are inconsistent in their completion of night-claim records. Both reliability and validity in a research method are capable of being checked and any research study should include plans to assess the likely accuracy and relevance of the methods which have been used to collect information.

In general, reliability is improved by better definition of procedures and criteria (which reduces observer errors) and is likely to be greater in prospective studies than retrospective studies. Validity is obviously reduced by unreliability, and further endangered by the introduction of observer or subject bias, which is particularly likely where interpretation as against observation of events is called for in the recording of information; and these biases are particularly liable to affect prospective studies.

Figure 7.3 summarises the main sources which may be used to collect research information and the brief notes which follow mention some of the strengths and limitations of each.

Figure 7.3: Methods of Collecting Information for Research

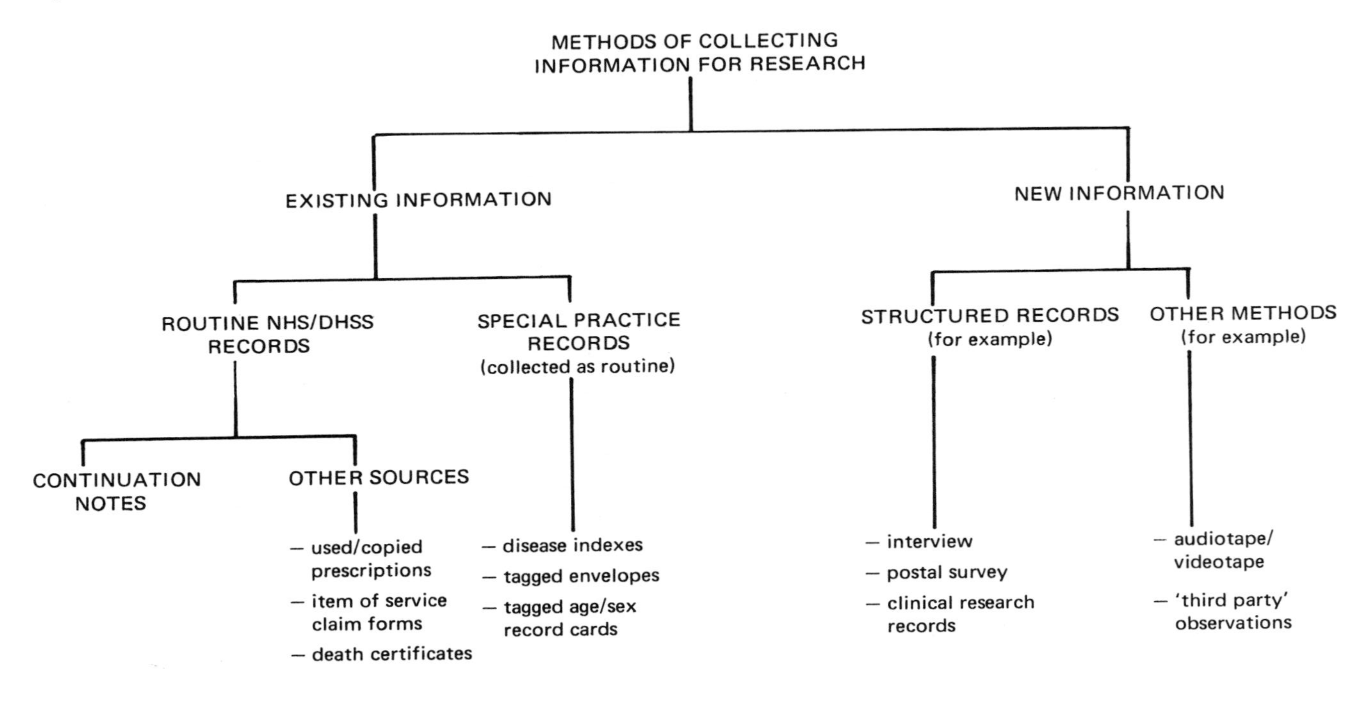

Continuation Notes in Routine Records

Routine practice records are understandably seen by many as the ideal source of information for general practice research. It is true that many years of history of the natural development of illness and its response to treatment may be contained in these records but unfortunately it is also true that these records are often incomplete, inaccurate and illegible. When one doctor is using his own records of patients always seen by himself the extent of these limitations will be known; but the more the patient has moved between doctors or between practices the more variable becomes the information. Are records made of home visits, of weekend and night calls? Are all prescribed drugs recorded? Do both partners record instructions regarding follow-up arrangements? What does one doctor mean by CVS-nil and another by migraine?

> Fry's properly cautious retrospective record based study (1975) of 87 hypertensives diagnosed in his practice between 1949 and 1959 and followed till 1974 shows the contribution and limitations of record-based research. Fry is unusual in having been able to look back to the early NHS years and find patients in whom records show '. . .a diastolic blood pressure of 100 mm.Hg or more. . .on. . .three occasions in a sitting position.' Almost the only events he comments on for this population are death, coronary artery disease and cardiac failure and his conclusions are general rather than specific: '. . .There is a group of individuals in whom the condition of hypertension is evidently benign and who will go on living for many years at terms with their high blood. pressures. . .'

Information from routine records must be used and interpreted with due regard to its uncertain reliability and thus its uncertain validity and quality.

Other Routinely Collected Information

Amongst the many routine forms which may form a basis for research are prescription forms (EC10, FP10), various claims for item-of-service payments ranging from immunisation to maternity claims, and death certificates. The validity and reliability of each varies in relation to the use to be made of the information.

> A study of one individual doctor's prescribing costs based on review of his numbered prescriptions during one month will only be valid if he is known to write only on his own forms and it is known that no one else has used his forms. As a means of costing the prescribing

> in a practice, the DHSS monthly audit method is valid; as a means of identifying the contribution of individual doctors it is invalid outside single-handed practice as the above sources of error are not corrected for.

The use of information on item-of-service claim forms may itself be valid, but the equation of claim forms with all items-of-service is not. It stands to reason that as maternity claims attract a relatively high fee, claims made will approximate closer to the total possible than will be the case in notification of infectious diseases where only a nominal fee is allowed. Similarly, the implications for doctor-patient relationships of asking patients to sign night-visit claims almost certainly influence the number of such claims made. The reliability of using night-visit claims as an indicator of night visits actually done is thus suspect, a point underestimated by Buxton *et al.* (1977) in their study of night visiting apparently by general practitioners.

The poor reliability of death certificates as an indicator of cause of death as against the event of death has long been known.

> In a study of 870 death certificates where the cause of death was certified as appendicitis or appendicectomy, further review of hospital records showed that in 65 deaths the patient had undergone surgery for some other major pathology which accounted for their symptoms. Death was related neither to appendicitis nor to appendicectomy. (Howie, 1966).

In summary, routine records may provide a useful source of research information, but in each case care has to be taken before accepting the quality of information as adequate. The research worker himself has a moral obligation in this respect as he is often best placed to recognise the weaknesses of the information he is proposing to use.

Special Routinely Collected Practice Records

In some practices, a diagnostic label is attached to all consultations and a disease index constructed as described earlier. Alternatively, selected conditions may be identified and age-sex record cards or record envelopes tagged accordingly (the Royal College of General Practitioners' tagging system is used in many practices). Once again the usefulness of such lists as a basis for research depends on the precision with which the conditions have been identified and the use to which the information is to be put.

> Madden (1977) attached stickers to the records of patients with a history of adverse drug reactions and was able to identify 263 patients in this category in his practice. Further study implicated a penicillin reaction in 183 patients and these patients formed the basis for a prospective survey of their allergic status.

One of the principal uses of indexes of this kind is the retrospective identification of patients for prospective study. The population for the further study has, of course, to be defined cautiously and will probably not be '*all* patients with "condition x" ' but rather 'a group of patients *all* of whom have or have had "condition x" '. This means of identifying patients for study may greatly reduce the time required to complete a research project – usually to the benefit of the project.

Structured Records

New information for research purposes is usually recorded on a specially designed record. Structured records, or questionnaires, can be administered by an interviewer, or self-administered by the respondent himself. They may be designed to collect exact information ('What is the temperature of the patient?') or more subjective information ('Is the patient depressed?'). And their design may be open-ended with questions allowing a wide range of answers ('Where would you seek advice regarding contraception?') or closed with a restricted range of options ('Would you seek contraceptive advice from your family doctor? – Yes/No').

Bennett & Ritchie's textbook *Questionnaires in Medicine* is a short and very readable book full of good advice on questionnaire design. The main warnings repeat the themes already stressed in this chapter; prefer simple to complex design and define the terms being used with as much precision and clarity as possible.

The purpose of the questions being asked should be clearly explained unless for some reason this seems inappropriate. Any questionnaire that loses the sympathy of the person completing it will be inaccurately, incompletely or even mischievously completed. If the respondent does not return or complete the document, interpretation of that non-response is crucial and becomes progressively more difficult as the percentage of no-returns rises.

The design and administration of a questionnaire should carefully avoid leading questions (that is, questions which suggest the answer wanted) and attempts should be made to check both the validity and reliability of the particular questionnaire used. In a number of clinical conditions, standard questionnaires, already tested and found valid and reliable, can be used (examples include the Medical Research Council questionnaire on respiratory symptoms, the Beck Depression Inventory, the Barker & Bishop thyroid follow-up questionnaire, all of which are described in detail in Bennett & Ritchie's book). Use of established methods not only saves time in designing and testing new forms but also increases the comparability of new and old work.

Where attempts are being made to measure objective attributes, questionnaires can be constructed in a relatively open manner without risking the collection of material which will prove difficult to analyse. The question

'IS THE PATIENT FEVERED : YES or NO'

allows the collection of much less information than the alternative

'WHAT IS THE TEMPERATURE : ________'

where replies can be sub-divided as required at a later stage, say into (i) 36-7°C, (ii) 37-8°C, (iii) 38-40°C and (iv) 40+°C.

However, in many general practice projects, the information being sought is more diffuse and subjective. The research worker will often want to be able to examine replies, using not only simple breakdowns of the 'present' or 'absent' variety, but also more discriminating analyses of gradations of the attitudes or opinions held by the responders. In this situation, leaving the opportunity to respond to questions 'open', risks the collection of replies which will be unacceptably difficult to categorise at a later stage. For the purposes of this kind of research, attitude and rating scales are particularly helpful.

For example:

IN REGARD TO USE OF COMMERCIAL DEPUTISING SERVICES, ARE YOU

STRONGLY IN FAVOUR	IN FAVOUR	UNDECIDED	AGAINST	STRONGLY AGAINST

The two outer columns on each side can be summated to provide a crude *for* and *against* figure; the finer sub-division offers a greater insight a into strengths of opinion.

Alternatively rating scales allow the ranking of attitudes or attributes; responders are asked to mark where on the scale (of ten points in the example below) their experience lies:

SINCE STARTING THESE TABLETS INDICATE HOW MUCH THE FOLLOWING SYMPTOMS OF YOUR ILLNESS HAVE IMPROVED OR GOT WORSE

	Improved	The same	Worse
ABILITY TO SLEEP	5	0	5
FEELING OF WELL-BEING	5	0	5
INTEREST IN WORK	5	0	5

A number of pieces of common sense advice should be kept in mind when sending out questionnaires. Include a courteous, simple but informative covering letter; unless quite out of the question enter the name of the recipient by hand and sign the letter personally; address the envelopes by hand and use postage stamps rather than franking machines. The introduction of this kind of personal touch is likely to increase the willingness of potential helpers to become involved. It is wise not to ask too many questions, or to make them too complicated. It is also essential to avoid using questions which include double negatives, and sensible to avoid offering options such as 'tick YES/NO' where a line through the YES could mean either YES or NO. Remember to include a reply-paid envelope where relevant; include a guarantee of confidentiality; offer feedback if possible and include some means of identifying who has responded and who has not. Finally, before using any questionnaire or research record, try it out personally and ask some friends or colleagues to comment on it and try it themselves.

Other Methods

Less conventional research methods include the use of audiotape or videotape and the use of an observer at the consultation. Audiotape recording has been used by Bain to examine consultations of his own (1976) and by Byrne & Long to record other doctors at work (1976). Although there is a real risk of observer bias when this kind of material is being analysed, the evidence remains available and the interpretations can be checked as required. The validity of the method becomes suspect only if recording interferes with the doctor's or the patient's behaviour during the consultation. Although audiotape recording is probably discreet enough for its presence to be forgotten about, videotape is usually more obtrusive and the validity of observations made using it less certain. The same applies to the use of an observer 'sitting-in' at a consultation. However, the presence of even these apparently major distractions can quickly be forgotten by both doctor and patient and much information of value obtained (Buchan & Richardson, 1973).

Direct observations have, of course, been used in workstudy in industry for many years and Floyd & Livesey (1975) have described a technique (bleep activity sampling) for recording how doctors use their time throughout the working week.

As research in general practice moves into the more difficult areas of behaviour and relationships it is likely that more use will have to be made of techniques which 'photograph' or reproduce relevant consultations, perhaps by simulation. The results of such work will inevitably arouse controversy and the onus lies on those experimenting with such methods to demonstrate their validity as measures of the realities of practice.

The Size of a Study

Deciding how large a study should be, how long it should last, and how many doctors should be asked to help, are important and often difficult decisions. Sometimes clear advice can be given, particularly on minimum requirements, but often only general guidelines can be offered.

Statistical Advice

Statistical help is almost unobtainable in some areas but readily accessible in others. The degree of support offered also varies, often reflecting the level of interest in medical research of the particular statistician. A helpful statistician will advise on many different aspects of the design and analysis of a research project, and when this service is available it may be possible to predict with some accuracy how many patients will have to be recruited for a particular question to be answered. But the doctor himself must do his own background thinking. He should know the expected incidence or prevalence of the main events in which he is interested and know the main characteristics of the population available to him for the study. He should have thought of the methods he might use and the probable accuracy of the information he will collect. He should also have decided what he would regard as clinically significant findings. No matter how good the statistician, the quality of his advice cannot be the best if this information is missing or inaccurate.

Expert advice is particularly necessary when clinical trials are being planned to ensure that the proposed design is capable of producing findings which will be statistically significant as well as clinically significant. Assurance that statistical advice has been taken is required by many funding agencies and such help is essential when very small numerators are expected or very large denominators likely.

General Guidelines

When expert advice is not being used, the first step is to think about the way the principal findings from the study will be tabulated. It is desirable that numbers presented in important sub-divisions of tables of results should be 20 or above, as figures below 10 will lead to difficulties in statistical testing.

> Freedman's (1976) study of breast feeding analyses 79 case histories. In all but one of the analyses presented, 20 or more patients are included. In one division patients are separated into primiparae (33) and multiparae (46). The multiparous patients are then divided into those who have previously breast fed (20) and those who have not (24). When analysing whether breast feeding was attempted in relation to social class, classes I and II were amalgamated as were classes IV and V, to ensure three socio-economic groupings with adequate numbers in each (23, 36 and 20). Had five groupings been wished, a larger study would almost certainly have been necessary.

Once the necessary number of events (for example, illnesses, consultations, or referrals) has been estimated, the number of practices which would produce these numbers, over various periods of time, can be calculated from information in the literature or from pilot studies or by making 'informed guesses'. The remaining dilemma is the choice on how to recruit the necessary size of patient population or sample. Either many doctors can be asked to contribute a few patients over a short time, or fewer doctors (or one doctor) can study more patients over a longer time.

Each policy has advantages and disadvantages. The more doctors who are involved, the greater the difficulty of ensuring standard criteria of recording and the greater the likelihood of losing co-operation over the duration of a study. The duration is itself an important consideration; the longer a study lasts, the more likely it is that 'time' itself will become a variable which will influence the results produced. From a different angle, most doctors can maintain interest in a project of their own choosing and design over a period of a year or more. But doctors co-operating in projects designed by others will usually require considerable motivation to produce any quantity of information for longer than six months; and epidemics, holidays and illnesses inevitably affect continuity of interest and thus involvement. Particular problems are created by studies which require long-term follow-up, and the difficulties of obtaining good-quality information over a long prospective study may be a justification for accepting the different but often comparable disadvantages of a retrospective study.

Sometimes the reasons for deciding on a particular size of a study may be more empirical: a month's review of an appointments system; a year's out-of hours calls; or the follow-up of 100 patients with otitis media. This approach is more likely to be adequate in purely descriptive studies and less likely to meet the demand of projects aiming to test even simple hypotheses.

Ethics in Research

The two ethical issues which cause most concern in general practice research are confidentiality (including the propriety of conducting surveys of populations either ill or well) and the use of controls or placebo-takers in therapeutic trials.

Several important reports have appeared in the *British Medical Journal* in recent years and are recommended reading for any doctor planning a research project. The World Medical Association's 'Declaration of Helsinki' (*British Medical Journal*, 1964) is too brief and too general although widely quoted. Two Medical Research Council reports cover clearly and comprehensively all the important dilemmas. The first of these reports 'Responsibility in Investigations on Human Subjects' (1964) comments separately on 'procedures contributing to the benefit of the individual patient', the use of 'control subjects in investigations of treatment or prevention' and 'procedures not of direct benefit to the individual'. The definition of 'informed consent' is discussed helpfully and the particular problems arising in research involving children are recognised. The more recent report 'Responsibility in the Use of Medical Information for Research' (1973) examines problems of confidentiality in relation to medical records and computers and discusses the ethical issues raised by different methods of collecting information. Some of these are particularly relevant to research in the community, whether by general practitioners, by other doctors or, most importantly, by non-medical personnel. Amongst the methods discussed are 'surveys of apparently well populations', 'research based wholly on medical records', 'research requiring access to subjects identified from medical records', and 'research involving access to relatives of patients'.

The main conclusions from these reports are first that the support of a responsible professional body should always be sought before research involving procedures on patients is started (an ethical committee's approval is indeed a prerequisite with some employing authorities and grant-giving bodies), and second that community-based studies, which involve patients registered with doctors who are not involved as collaborators in the study, should be referred to a local medical committee or its equivalent for discussion and approval.

The onus on the individual research planner to design ethically acceptable research remains a legal as well as a moral responsibility. Campbell's essay 'Infants, Children and Informed Consent' (1974) balances the risks of inhibiting worthwhile research by over-strict interpretation of ethical codes against the need to protect patients from unacceptable procedures. His conclusion that the integrity of the investigator is an important part of safeguarding against unethical research is as full of insight as it is simple.

The only further point I wish to make relates to the ethics of the use of 'controls' in clinical trials and the possibility that double-blind designs may infringe the doctor-patient relationship which is central to good medical care. Clinical trials which compare a new drug with the best drug available at the time or with a placebo if no treatment is known to be effective, appear at least as ethically acceptable as the use of any other measure (new or old) which has not been fully evaluated. If it is accepted as wrong to become involved in inadequate research which may produce results so weighted by subjective factors and other errors of design as to be invalid, then the choice comes to lie between doing no research or using controls or placebos in a proper 'double-blind' manner. The solution to this problem will not always be the same.

In Summary

By now it should be possible to commit some reasonably definite proposals to paper. A full statement of research proposals and plans will include:

introduction and review of literature;
aims of study;
methods of collecting information;
methods proposed for analysis of results;
financial requirements;
technical details of specialised procedures;
recording forms to be used;
references;
curriculum vitae of research worker.

There are several uses to which the full statement (often referred to as a 'research protocol') may be put and the details of the statement will vary accordingly. An application for funding will include all items listed above whereas a request for support from an ethical committee need not discuss financial requirements and may omit, for example, the finer details on methods of collecting and analysing information. A statement for colleagues who have agreed to collaborate in collecting information may include little more than instructions on how to collect relevant information.

The section on methods of collecting information is the most important part of the document. The main 'events' to be studied should be clearly stated and defined. The population to be studied must be described in detail and a full statement included on how any samples are to be drawn. Conditions for exclusions from the sample may be stated. Instructions and explanatory information to be given to patients and other staff involved in the study should be explicit.

Instructions on who to contact in the case of difficulties – which almost always arise – should be stated and guarantees of confidentiality given (and honoured!).

A research statement should be short and general enough to be read quickly and clearly by a busy external assessor not necessarily expert in the particular field, but at the same time detailed enough to act as a precise guide to the methods to be used and to demonstrate that adequate attention has been given to the details of design already described in this chapter. From introduction to analysis of results the text should not normally exceed 2,000 words. No statement should be finalised until it has been criticised by someone qualified to give an opinion on its adequacy and appropriateness.

References

Bain, D.J.G., 'Doctor-patient Communication in General Practice Consultations', *British Journal of Medical Education*, 10 (1976), pp.125-31.

Bennett, A.E. & Ritchie, K., *Questionnaires in Medicine* (Oxford University Press, London, 1975).

Buchan, I.C. & Richardson, I.M., 'Time Study of Consultations in General Practice', *Scottish Health Service Studies*, no.27 (Scottish Home & Health Department, 1973).

Buxton, M.J., Klein, R.E. & Sayers, J., 'Variations in GP Night-visiting Rates, Medical Organisation and Consumer Demand', *British Medical Journal*, 1 (1977), pp.827-30.

Byrne, P.S. & Long, B.E.L., *Doctors Talking to Patients*, Department of Health & Social Security (HMSO, London, 1976).

Campbell, A.G.M., 'Infants, Children and Informed Consent', *British Medical*

Journal, 3 (1974), pp.334-8.

Eimerl, T.S. & Laidlaw, A.J., *A Handbook for Research in General Practice* (Livingstone, London, 1969).

Everett, M.T., 'The Place of Antibiotics in the Treatment of Acute Gastro-enteritis in General Practice: a Controlled Trial', *Journal of the Royal College of General Practitioners*, 23 (1973), pp.183-93.

Floyd, C.B. & Livesey, A., 'Self-observation in General Practice – the Bleep Method', *Journal of the Royal College of General Practitioners*, 25 (1975), pp.425-31.

Freedman, G.R., 'Breast Feeding – a Year's Experience of One Group Practice', *Journal of the Royal College of General Practitioners*, 26 (1976), pp.507-13.

Fry, J., 'Deaths and Complications from Hypertension', *Journal of the Royal College of General Practitioners*, 25 (1975), pp.489-94.

Howie, J.G.R., 'Death from Appendicitis and Appendicectomy', *Lancet*, 2 (1966), pp.1334-7.

Madden, T.A., 'Adverse Penicillin Reactions in the Records of a General Practice 1973-5', *Journal of the Royal College of General Practitioners*, 27 (1977), pp.73-7.

Medical Research Council, 'Responsibility in Investigations on Human Subjects', *British Medical Journal*, 2 (1964), pp.178-80.

Medical Research Council, 'Responsibility in the Use of Medical Information for Research', *British Medical Journal*, 1 (1973), pp.213-16.

Royal College of General Practitioners, 'A General Practice Glossary', *Journal of the Royal College of General Practitioners*, 23 supplement 3 (1973).

Royal College of General Practitioners, *Oral Contraceptives and Health* (Whitefriars Press, London, 1974).

Westcott, R., 'Consultation Length in General Practice', *Journal of the Royal College of General Practitioners*, 27 (1977), pp.552-5.

Witts, L.J., *Medical Surveys and Clinical Trials* (Oxford University Press, London, 1964).

World Medical Association, 'Declaration of Helsinki', *British Medical Journal*, 2 (1964), p.177.

8 FUNDING RESEARCH

Part of planning a project involves working out its likely costs and thinking about how these are to be met. Many good projects cost nothing more than pen and paper plus, of course, research worker's time. At the other end of the scale are projects which require the employment of full-time staff and the support of expensive information-processing resources, and these absorb the larger part of the £1 million (at 1975 prices) which is available each year for research in general practice or by general practitioners. Most of the projects which service general practitioners design lie nearer the inexpensive end of this spectrum. However, finding sums of money of no more than two or three hundred pounds can be surprisingly difficult and projects may have to be reduced in scale to a level which can be met by available practice personnel and income. This chapter looks briefly at how to cost a project and how to absorb modest expenses without seeking independent funding, at where to look for any funds required and at some of the technical and tactical aspects of applying for a grant.

Costing a Project

Costs can be calculated under the headings personnel, materials, travelling and processing of results.

Personnel

Research requires time; time for design, for fieldwork, for analysis of results and for writing about the results, and much of this is usually provided as voluntary overtime by those most interested in the research. There are, however, three ways in which an allowance for doctors' time may be included in claims for funds. The first is the full-time or part-time research fellow; the second is the sessional payment to the doctors organising the work to enable them to buy time – and thus co-operation and goodwill – from the partnerships involved in the research; the third is the item-of-service payment, for example, for patients contributed, or questionnaires completed by doctors helping with the project. When costing the first method, the claim should be in line with national scales for appropriately qualified personnel and allow for employers' superannuation and national insurance contributions and incremental payments as appropriate. The second method of claiming is more likely to succeed when the financing body has requisitioned the study and the third method, which is more controversial, begs the question of whether quantity of information can be purchased without sacrifice of quality (*Sunday Times*, 1978).

Since professional non-medical personnel can play an invaluable role in collecting research information, sessional employment of nurses, health visitors and those trained in sociology or social work may be worth considering. Practices are, of course, reimbursed for employment of nursing (and secretarial) staff up to agreed levels and a limited amount of slack time may unofficially be used for collecting research information. Because research aims to contribute to improved patient care, this use of health service resources seems to me to be morally justifiable. Using the same argument it seems reasonable to set modest non-reimbursable costs against income tax as an expense of the practice.

Secretarial help is often an important part of successful research. Separate assessment should be made of the help which will be required to construct the project, of the time which will be needed during the fieldwork, and of the work which will be involved in subsequent analysis of data and presentation of results. Once again rates of pay should reflect national salary scales. Unduly high or low rates may create frictions which will affect both the clinical and the research work of the practice team. Before deciding on conditions of employment, implications of various hourly 'contracts' for insurance and taxation purposes should be discussed with the personnel involved.

Materials

Grant applications frequently differentiate between capital outlays (which will outlast the research) and expendable items (which will be used up during the project). Major capital outlays generally refer to items like centrifuges, incubators and microscopes, which are not likely to figure prominently in a general practice project, although items such as filing cabinets, calculators, tape recorders and typewriters would also fall within this category. Expendable items will include costs for postages, stationery, printing and telephone. Allowance should be made for possible rises in postal costs and, when questionnaires are being used, include the cost of sending reminders and paying for posting of replies. Where high response rates are anticipated, the use of pre-stamped reply-cards (or envelopes) is justified; when response rates are likely to be low, money can be saved by using the business reply-card system for which the cost is determined by the number of cards returned together with surcharge. Details on how to obtain and use the business reply-card can be had through the Post Office. Many university departments (and the Royal College of General Practitioners) hold business reply licences and may be willing to act as 'post office' for individual research projects. Thought should be given to printing rather than duplicating or photocopying questionnaires or circulars. Printing is a relatively inexpensive extra outlay which can transform the image projected by research from amateur to professional. Commercial services are more expensive than those available through universities and estimates of cost should be made before commissioning such work.

Travelling

Estimated costs of car travel, for example, to recruit doctors, to visit patients or to deliver specimens, and of payments to patients who are asked to travel for the purposes of the research, will normally be included under a separate heading in a grant application. Many funding bodies recognise the importance of helping research workers to meet colleagues or experts working in the same field and are willing to meet rather non-specific estimated outlays for 'travel'. However, the cost of travel to present results at meetings normally has to be met from other sources.

Data Processing

I have placed this item separately to emphasise its importance. Many general practitioners receiving support from a university department or from a Royal College of General Practitioners Research Unit may be given access to data processing help without charge. When this is the case, the projects should be designed to fit with those resources that are already available as, for example, the adapting of computer programmes not only depends on scarce personnel being available, but may take months of work rather than days. Frequently very small studies will be supported free under the umbrella of large projects. More ambitious projects may be required to contribute to certain aspects of the cost of data processing (punch cards, operator's time, computer files – all reasonably inexpensive) but excused from having to meet the much higher costs of computer time. Costing the data processing needs of major projects is beyond the scope of this book.

Sources of Research Money

Money for research is provided principally through state funds (Department of Health and Social Security, Regional Health Authorities and Hospital Endowments, Scottish Home and Health Department,

University Grants Committee, Medical Research Council), through a large number of voluntary organisations (including, for example, the Nuffield Provincial Hospitals Trust, the Multiple Sclerosis Society, the Leukaemia Research Fund) and through the Pharmaceutical Industry. *The Research Funds Guide* issued by the British Medical Association gives a comprehensive, though not complete, list of bodies (including more than 90 voluntary organisations) to whom application can be made (BMA, 1976).

Deciding where to apply may be difficult, and it is worth taking advice from colleagues who have first-hand information about the availability of money locally, or nationally. Often there are local trusts or funds earmarked for research and the general practitioner looking for a small amount of money may attract support from these. Allocations from national funds are more difficult to secure and long delays in receiving decisions are common, as is failure to attract support despite presentation of apparently sound projects. Clearly voluntary bodies tend to support the research interests implied by their titles and, in the same way, pharmaceutical companies tend to support projects in which they can identify possible value from a commercial viewpoint.

State funds are used to:

promote research in areas identified from time to time as priorities (for example, incontinence, geriatric care, dyspepsia);

balance investment between fundamental research into the nature of disease and applied research into the application of existing knowledge to health service organisation;

support the examination of new concepts which may have a wider general application to medical progress; and

help individual research workers (established or new) who appear to have potential which should be supported.

Overall policy is outlined by the chief scientist organisations and applied by the various funding sub-committees according to their titles. Much time can be wasted by applying to the wrong committee and it is always wise to ask the secretary of any trust or fund, to which an application is being considered, whether the project falls within the scope and scale of the funds available. Major applications may be refused by, for example, a Regional Health Authority, because they feel the project should be within the remit of the Medical Research Council; and, in turn, the MRC might decline support because they are already supporting similar work elsewhere in the country.

General practitioners are particularly likely to receive support from the Scientific Foundation Board of the Royal College of General Practitioners. Several thousand pounds are available annually, usually for distribution in packages of under £1,000, and often to doctors wanting to mount 'pilot' studies which might provide a basis for a later application to other sources. Once again, advice should be sought from the officers of the Foundation before making formal application.

The College offers a number of awards for proposed, current or even completed research. The Mackenzie prize of £1,000 is awarded every five years, generally for completed research. Annual awards such as the Ian Dingwall Grant prize (for doctors up to 36 years of age), the Ian Stokoe prize (for research involving the use of illustration) and the Astra prizes (for trainees) are smaller, but none the lesss useful, sources of money.

Applying for Money

The advice on how to apply for money which is given in the opening three pages of the BMA *Research Funds Guide* (referred to above) cannot easily be bettered and should be read and followed by all applicants for research money. The main rules are:

apply in good time;
apply to the right body;
think the project out thoroughly before drawing up the application,
and do not be deterred if your application is turned down.

Many bodies have standard instructions as to how applications should be presented and to disregard these invites delay and implies a carelessness which might be regarded as inappropriate in a potential researcher.

The normal format for a grant application is along the lines described on page 86. Reference should be made to any specialist collaboration which has been arranged (for laboratory or radiological or statistical services, for example) and any experts who have advised on the design of the study may be named, if this seems appropriate.

The applicant should include a *curriculum vitae*, stating his current occupation and the previous posts he has held, describing other relevant experience in clinical or research work, and listing any published work.

The application should be concise and at the same time readable and any references to the literature should be double-checked for accuracy at their original sources – the effect of sending assessors to look up non-existent references needs little elaboration!

The application should state whether the approval of an ethical committee has been sought and obtained. Other sources of funding which are currently being explored should be listed; a note of unsuccessful approaches made may either help or hinder an application and the best policy on this particular issue will vary from application to application.

As with a paper prepared for submission to a journal, first drafts should be left and revised after a reasonable interval, and should also be read and criticised by at least two colleagues with different backgrounds. Often the names of members of grant-giving bodies are known and it is generally regarded as appropriate that their advice be sought before an application is submitted. This is sensible as it may allow weaknesses to be identified and particularly appropriate slants to be emphasised. Canvassing members of committees after the application has been made is inadvisable.

Administration of a Grant. Small grants (under £1,000) may be administered by the applicant through his practice accounts or a savings account opened for the purposes of the project. Where larger sums are involved and, in particular, when full-time salaries are payable, it should be clear whether the sums asked for represent only gross salaries required, or include necessary extras for employers' contributions to superannuation and national insurance. Grant-giving bodies may wish major awards to be administered by a formal institution – such as a university. Many administering bodies request a fixed percentage (around 10 per cent) to cover overheads and some grant-giving bodies ask this to be included in the application, while others negotiate it later.

If the costs of a research project can be met from readily available resources, use them. Time is saved and the risk of having the disappointment of an application being rejected is avoided. If money has to be found elsewhere, take time to ensure that the application is properly prepared, and submit it to a body likely to offer support. Money *is* available for good general practice research, and both the need and opportunity for research in general practice are widely recognised.

Research Funds Guide, British Medical Association 3rd edn. (BMA, London, 1976).
Sunday Times, 29 January 1978, p.4.

9 ORGANISING THE WORK

Even with a good research idea and a soundly designed research plan, success is not invariable. The dividing line between satisfactory and unsatisfactory outcome is often fine, described as luck by those who fail and judgement by those who succeed. The aim of this short chapter is to emphasise, and in some cases re-emphasise, the importance of paying attention to a number of superficially obvious but often neglected aspects of the organisation of research.

In the next chapter, which traces the development of the research ideas I introduced in Chapter 6, the practical implications of spending time on these issues will be seen more clearly. Organisation can be thought of under the headings 'before fieldwork', 'during fieldwork' and 'after fieldwork'.

Before Fieldwork

Timing

Research almost always takes longer to plan than expected. It is important to allow for this and at the same time realise that there are good and bad times to start and carry out research. A study of respiratory illness, for example, may run short of material in June, have plenty in November – and too much in January! The summer is usually less satisfactory for research than the winter, and holiday times are generally inconvenient either because of extra practice commitments or other distractions.

After deciding when the fieldwork should start and how long it is likely to take, make plans which allow for additional time beforehand in which to try out methods, arrange assistance and make final administrative arrangements.

Recruiting and Explanation

Recruiting helpers (whether research subjects or assistants) from amongst one's patients or colleagues is often an essential part of preliminary organisation. Here the dilemma lies between defining a population for study and finding that the selected patients or doctors don't wish to take part, and on the other hand recruiting willing helpers but then having difficulty finding their common denominator when attempting to describe who or what they represent. People you know and have an empathy with are more likely to participate as requested than are strangers or those you know to be unsympathetic to you or to the aims of your inquiry; patients of unstable background or low intelligence are less likely to comply with instructions than are those with more insight. In short, as far as is compatible with sound research design, those doctors and patients more rather than less likely to help, should be enlisted.

Both patients and doctors should be given time to think over a request for help. A letter explaining the general aims of a study linked with a request to be allowed to explain more of the details at a later time is better than a snap request for a yes/no decision over the telephone, in the surgery, or at a meeting. This tends to produce initial 'yes' answers but be associated with drop-outs at a later stage; the first approach on the other hand may produce more initial 'no' answers but yields a greater eventual return from those who do agree to participate. Requests for help should include a stamped envelope or card for reply or indicate when and how a further approach will be made. Offers of help made by doctors when in their own premises, or by patients in their own homes, are more likely to be honoured than those made on neutral ground or on the 'territory' of the organiser of the project.

When either doctors or patients are being enlisted as helpers it is important to give informative explanations of the proposed research. Sometimes the design of the study necessitates withholding full details to prevent the risk of introducing observer or subject bias. Each individual researcher must make his own moral decision on where to draw the line between spoiling the research by giving complete information and misleading one's helpers by incomplete truth. My own aim has been to strike whatever compromise will ensure that at the end of any study colleagues or patients will feel that their trust in my motives as a research worker has not been misplaced and that they would help again at a later date if asked. The issues of 'informed consent' are particularly important when patients are asked to take drugs, give blood or undergo investigation. Leaflets, approved by an independent adviser or ethical committee, explaining the reasons for such research and outlining any procedures involved should be available for all patients concerned. Professional colleagues participating in a study will of course receive an appropriate statement of the aims and methods of the study.

Production of Material

I have already discussed the preparation of material to be used during a research study. Printing is more attractive than duplication of typewriting, real stamps are more personal than office frankings, neatly parcelled drug or investigation kits more impressive than loose unlabelled bottles and handwritten signatures immensely more personal than fake signatures – which are even worse when done in different colours to look real! Research is still a part of the doctor-patient contract in its widest sense and is enhanced by observation of the same personal courtesies which apply at the consultation. Indeed, one of the differences between good and second-rate research often appears to be the care taken to market it professionally.

Specialist Support

The support of a statistician should have been enlisted by now, and experts in data handling feel that they too should advise on research before rather than during or after the fieldwork. However, my reference to this topic here relates specifically to colleagues whose help is required for laboratory, radiological or other opinions. Their active support should be sought not only out of courtesy but also because their particular knowledge may lead to improvement of the research design. Bacteriological assessments of improperly taken specimens and radiological opinions on inappropriate films are literally worse than useless. Remember too that nursing colleagues, secretaries, receptionists and patients are also experts within their own fields; if they are to be involved, ask for their support rather than take it for granted, explain the aims of your study and listen to criticisms and advice.

Interest and involvement foster co-operation and success.

Pilot Studies

Many research experts regard a pilot study as an essential part of any research enterprise. My own preference has always been to rely more on discussions of detail with colleagues than on doing actual pilot studies; but I do advise asking friends to try out any questionnaires to be used and would always keep open the option of discarding the first week or so of recording in a study if modification of design proves advisable.

During Fieldwork

Checking Progress

While information is being collected it is highly desirable to be able to check on whether the intentions and details of the methods are being observed. If they are not, attempt to identify whether the difficulties are due to the design of the project, or due to mistakes by the participants or, as is usually the case, come from a mixture of the two. Correct faults in the design and attempt to clarify sources of possible confusion.

As well as checking on the completion of forms and records, make some preliminary analyses of the results as they come in. Often, for example, trends in the early and later replies to a questionnaire can be compared and differences which may aid interpretation of the significance of non-responses can be identified. Check whether the quantity of material is matching expectations, whether some participants are providing more material than others and whether necessary and expected differences between groups seem likely to be achieved. Be prepared to drop unsatisfactory parts of the study, to prolong or shorten the study and to recruit more helpers if the aims of the study require and are compatible with this. Where defaulters or non-responders can be identified arrange for follow-up. Most who are going to reply to a circular do so by return of post and few replies will be received later than two weeks after the mailing. Then is the time for any reminders proposed. Ambiguous answers should be clarified, unexpected outcomes or side-effects monitored and necessary action discussed and taken. The fieldwork period may be one of relative inactivity; but only if progress is known to be as satisfactory as can be achieved!

Personnel Management

Keep the participants' feeling of interest and involvement high by discussing the project by personal contact, telephone or letter. If a project is to last six months, give a progress report at three months, not necessarily discussing results – as this might introduce bias – but saying, for example, what level of response has been achieved and what remains to be done. Indicate difficulties which have appeared (before the three months had elapsed if they are important) and thank colleagues for their support.

After Fieldwork

As soon as the fieldwork is concluded, decide how to thank your helpers, and think about what information you can return to them. Sometimes response will have been anonymous and then feedback and thanks are not possible. If results are likely to be available within say three months one communication may be enough but, particularly if the number of helpers has been few, think of sending an immediate letter of thanks, a later note of results, and eventually a reprint of any publication. Once again this is partly common courtesy, but also helps demonstrate the value of the help that has been given and may encourage willingness to help on some future occasion. Remember that helpers may include patients as well as colleagues; and lay colleagues as well as professional colleagues.

The basic lessons are simple. Good organisation requires:

adequate time, particularly for planning;
willingness to consult those likely to be able to help and to be involved by the research;
flexibility to change and adapt plans if necessary during the fieldwork.

10 SIX PROJECTS

In the last three chapters I have outlined the more important principles of research design and illustrated some of these with examples from the literature of general practice. The ideal and the practical are not always the same and in this chapter I want to show some of the ways in which difficulties arise and how compromises are made. I will do this by describing the studies which were designed to explore the research interests introduced in Chapter 6. After a brief reminder of the thinking behind each project, each study is summarised using the profile:

NUMERATOR (OR EVENTS)
DENOMINATOR (OR POPULATION/SAMPLE)
TYPE OF STUDY
METHODS OF COLLECTING INFORMATION
SIZE OF STUDY
ETHICS
FUNDING
ORGANISATION

After presenting this outline I will discuss why some of these decisions on design were taken and why some were probably correct, but others wrong.

Project One: 'Early or Late Antibiotics in a Flu Epidemic?' (continued from page 52).

Faced with uncertainty as to whether respiratory illnesses presenting during outbreaks of 'influenza' should be treated routinely with antibiotics, a colleague and myself (each partners in separate but neighbouring practices of three doctors and 6,000 patients) set out to compare the outcomes of early treatment of influenza-like illnesses with a tetracycline on the one hand and a placebo on the other hand.

The study was designed thus:

NUMERATOR — outcome to be measured in (i) number of days in each illness where any of the following symptoms were present: cough, spit, purulent spit, purulent nasal discharge; (ii) attendances

	at the doctor, time off work with or without a certificate and (iii) side effects attributed to tablets taken.
DENOMINATOR	male volunteers, aged between 18 and 50, whose occupation, family and domestic setting would be known and whose stated smoking habits would be recorded; and suffering from any self-diagnosed cold or influenza-like illness which was not settling spontaneously after 48 hours and which would then be treated using the trial medication (patients with chronic respiratory illness and any other serious long-term illness were excluded later, as were patients with any drug allergy).
TYPE OF STUDY	prospective double-blind clinical trial during six winter months using patients as described under 'denominator' randomly allocated to takers of antibiotic (demethyl-chlortetracycline) or of matched placebo.
METHOD OF COLLECTING INFORMATION	patients' self-recorded responses on appropriately designed cards.
SIZE OF STUDY	as many patients as were willing to take part from the two practices (total population 12,000); six months (November to April) and all treated illnesses during that time.
ETHICS	because disagreement existed on whether antibiotics are needed for flu-like illnesses, comparison of active against placebo in double-blind random controlled trial setting appeared ethically acceptable.
FUNDING	a pharmaceutical company was willing to provide all necessary drugs suitably packaged, to finance all printing and postage and to finance 15 hours' secretarial help weekly for one year.
ORGANISATION	discussed below.

Two difficulties outside our control and one of our own making had to be overcome. The first difficulty was that four of the six partners in the two practices, although willing to co-operate in the study, expressed understandable concern regarding extra work during an epidemic; the design had to make minimum demands on doctors' time or risk loss of support which could compromise the main intentions of the study. The solution to this problem appeared to be to arrange that all assessments of progress be made by the patients themselves and to accept the absence of information from physical examination, except where recorded in clinical notes of patients consulting. The second problem, overlapping in some aspects, concerned the clinical grounds for entry to the study. Given that decisions to consult with minor respiratory illness often bear little relationship to the severity of the illness and that a patient's assessment of a flu-like illness is often of as much diagnostic significance as is the doctor's assessment, it seemed reasonable to allow patients to make their own decision to start a course of treatment – within, of course, guidelines provided as part of the instructions for the study. This had the advantage of removing the risk of doctor-bias in selection of illnesses for inclusion (and exclusion) and also removing the risk of doctor-bias in assessing the stage the illness had reached when treatment was started. The acceptability of these solutions to the two problems depended on patients adhering to the instructions they were given, both about initiating treatment and about reporting their progress, and the validity of the study became dependent on clear instructions and adequate compliance.

The third problem was determining the size of the study. With no real idea of the details of the likely morbidity of the next season's winter epidemic, no clear idea of the difference in outcome between the treated and placebo groups which was either to be expected or would be regarded as clinically significant, and no experience of how many patients would be willing to help as requested, we opted out completely from estimating the necessary or ideal size of the study. Our decision to opt for a six-month study, running from November to April, covered the most likely period for a flu epidemic, but none the less we were depending on luck rather than judgement in the crucial aspect of deciding the quantity of material required; female patients were excluded because we wished not to prescribe tetracycline unwittingly to those who might become pregnant, and because we wished to measure work loss as an indicator of outcome; the decision to study the age group 18-50 years was taken to exclude older patients in whom concurrent illness was more likely. Patients with drug allergy and, for example, chronic chest illness were asked in a subsequent letter to notify the doctors organising the study and were excluded from further participation.

Recruitment was started in April, six months before the hoped-for starting date of the trial. Male patients in the age group concerned were sent the letter shown in Figure 10.1; the date and the patient's name were entered by hand and the letter signed personally. No age-sex register existed in either practice and sorting through the record cards and addressing envelopes took most free evenings for about four weeks. Some 3,000 letters were sent out; one-third of the patients were not traced at the addresses on their record envelopes and just under 1,000 of the remaining 2,000 patients agreed to help. It quickly became clear that to have 1,000 patients attending two surgeries 'at a convenient time' in September or October was unrealistic; instead, two weeks before the study was due to start, each volunteer was posted a package containing:

tablets for two courses of either antibiotic or placebo;
six labelled cards on which to record his clinical progress during the six months of the study, already stamped for posting (Figure 10.2);
a letter of instruction regarding use of the tablets (Figure 10.3);
a covering explanatory letter (again addressed and signed personally); and
a 'registration card' for recording age, smoking habits and a number of personal details which were later to be used to check the comparability of test and control groups.

Return of the 'registration card' was regarded as indicating participation in the trial and 852 patients entered the study. All reply cards were identified by number and not by the patient's name.

Randomisation of numbered treatment packs between test and control groups was handled by the pharmaceutical company and packs were allocated to the patients after listing their names alphabetically; ampicillin had been agreed as the treatment for any patient requiring 'additional' antibiotic treatment during the study and I held a note of the treatment allocations were it felt necessary to break the code (this was not in fact done at any time).

A married lady with previous secretarial experience was engaged on a year's part-time basis starting three months before the collection of clinical data; although the necessary printed material was ordered three months in advance, it arrived only just in time, having had to be reprinted after it was discovered that two batches of January cards and no February cards had been printed; we almost overlooked the printing

Figure 10.1: Letter to Patients Inviting Participation in the Proposed Clinical Trial

14 Apsley Street,
GLASGOW. W. 1.

Dear,

Next winter we are hoping to compare two different approaches to the treatment of the common cold and 'flu-like illnesses in this and one of our neighbouring Practices.

Patients who agree to take part in the trial will be given tablets to take in the event of their catching a cold or "the 'flu" and they will be asked to record the results by ticking the appropriate parts of a pre-paid reply card. No examinations, X-rays, or blood tests will be carried out as part of this study. Taking part should thus cause almost no inconvenience and we hope might even mean shorter periods of illness with colds than is the average at present.

In all, we hope that just over 1,000 people will help in this study and this means that we hope that about three out of four people receiving this letter will agree to take part.

If you are willing to be one of the 1,000 please complete and return the enclosed post-card. Those taking part will be asked to attend the Surgery at a convenient time in September or October to collect their supplies of tablets and to have the details of the scheme explained.

All results will, of course, be treated as confidential.

We hope you will agree to help in this study which should give useful results to help reduce the inconvenience of the minor illnesses which trouble us all each winter.

Yours sincerely,

J. G. R. HOWIE.

Dr. CHRISTIE
Dr. HOWIE
Dr. WRIGHT

Figure 10.2: Card Issued to Volunteers to Self-record Information During January of Study

Code № 852 Treatment No:- 415 Month:-January

Date:	1	2	3	4	5	6	7	8	9	10	11	12	13	14	15	16	17	18	19	20	21	22	23	24	25	26	27	28	29	30	31
√Tick if you have a cold																													√	√	√
√Tick if you are off work with this																															
√Tick if you have a panel line for this																															
√Tick if you have a cough																															√
√Tick if you produce a spit																															√
√Tick if the spit is yellow or green																															√
√Tick if you have a yellow or green discharge from the nose																															√
√Tick if you attend your doctor																															
√Tick if you took trial tablets																															√

If you have taken a course of trial tablets have you had any side effects? Yes/No

If Yes, please describe:-

Please describe any other medicine you have taken for a cold or flu this month?

PLEASE POST ON LAST DAY OF MONTH IF POSSIBLE

Figure 10.3: Notes on Use of Trial Medication

THE TRIAL TABLETS.

If you feel at any time between 1st November and 30th April that you have caught a cold or have taken 'flu please follow these instructions.

1) As closely as possible to 48 hours from noticing that you are unwell, unless you feel that you are already almost recovered, start the course of tablets in one of the enclosed bottles.

2) Having started the course take one tablet every 12 hours - 8 a.m. and 8 p.m., for example - until the bottle is finished.

3) At the end of the course of ten tablets your course of treatment is finished. DO NOT start the second bottle. It is for use if you develop a second episode at a later period of the winter.

4) If you start a course, please finish it unless advised medically to the contrary.

5) If both your courses of treatment have been used please let us know and a further bottle will be issued to you.

Both bottles are identical and either may be used first. Please do not use both at once, and please do not use the tablets for your relatives and friends.

IMPORTANT:

If at any time you wish medical advice for your cold or 'flu, please request this exactly as before, but mention to the doctor that you are taking part in this study as this may influence your treatment.

No provision has been made in this study for the use of "cough bottles". Please use these or not as you would normally do. If you do use one please let us know on the appropriate reply card giving the name of the mixture if you know it, but if not, a note of its colour and consistency.

If at any time you are in doubt about how to use the tablets, please do not hesitate to ask for advice.

KEEP THE TABLETS OUT OF REACH OF

CHILDREN.

of reminder cards for sending to those failing to return their monthly progress cards, and this was eventually done during the first week of the study proper.

The detailed preparation of the study now paid off. In the end, the design had become extremely simple in concept. The doctors organising the study found the winter months took on a quite new interest and appeal despite a major influenza outbreak which indeed provided the necessary luck which we felt we had earned by otherwise careful planning. The patients responded magnificently by sending in 4,852 progress cards (92 per cent of the possible total) over 70 per cent without reminders, and taking over 800 courses of treatment. Our research secretary and the receptionists in the two practices became equally involved and before long it was clear that the massive response was making eventual success probable. (The results of this trial are presented on page 155 of Chapter 13.)

Project Two: 'Do "Diagnoses" Determine or Justify Management Decisions?' (continued from page 54)

The question 'How central is the making of a traditional "diagnosis" to general practice decisions on management?' led to proposing the hypothesis that a better correlation would be found between *clinical information collected* and *treatment given* than between either *clinical information collected* and *diagnosis made* or *diagnosis made* and *treatment given* in at least the field of antibiotic prescribing and respiratory illness. The profile of the project designed to test this hypothesis was as follows:

NUMERATOR	(i) 'diagnosis made' – a free choice of label/diagnosis was open to the doctor completing the form used for the study (Figure 10.4); (ii) 'treatment given' – a range of options for the doctor to complete; (iii) 'information collected' – mainly statements on symptoms and signs volunteered by patients or elicited by doctors, whether positive or negative.
DENOMINATOR	new consultations for respiratory illness during the second week of each month from November to April of the winter of study; consecutive consultations where feasible with a request to describe at least 20, and not more than 35,

	during any one recording sequence. 65 doctors were approached of whom 63 agreed to take part; the doctors were chosen mainly because they were known to me and already involved in student teaching.
TYPE OF STUDY	prospective.
METHODS OF COLLECTING INFORMATION	completion of questionnaire.
SIZE OF STUDY	the original hope was that 50 doctors would each contribute 100 consultations over six months giving 5,000 forms to analyse. To prove the hypothesis did not require the demonstration of any particular degree of difference between groups of observations and no specific size of study was thus required.
ETHICS	neither patient nor doctor was identified on the form. Confidentiality of patient-information was safeguarded by the doctor responsible for the patient; confidentiality of doctor-information was my responsibility.
FUNDING	an application for funds to the Scottish Advisory Committee for Medical Research was turned down; officially no reasons can be given. This delayed the study for one year. A grant to cover stationery and part-time secretarial help for one year was given by a pharmaceutical company.
ORGANISATION	see below.

The first of three potential weaknesses of this design was the risk of collecting inadequate or inaccurate numerator information through use of an invalid questionnaire. The design of the questionnaire gave opportunities to answer both closed and open questions and to tick responses or add detail as preferred. Formidable as the form appeared, the doctors were asked only to enter clinical information which had influenced their handling of the consultation and specifically requested not to ask extra questions or carry out extra examination. Each doctor was given a supply of forms to try out before the project started and it

Figure 10.4: Questionnaire for Collecting Information on New Consultations for Respiratory Illness

RESPIRATORY ILLNESS IN GENERAL PRACTICE - PRESENTING SYMPTOMS AND SIGNS

CODE NUMBER:

1. PATIENT COMPLAINTS

	Tick ✓ Yes	Tick ✓ No	If 'yes', for how long
"THE COLD"			
"FLU"			
VAGUELY UNWELL			
LOSS OF APPETITE			
VOMITING			
DIARRHOEA			
CRYING			
HEADACHE			
SORE EARS			
SORE THROAT			
HOARSENESS			
COUGH			
NIGHT COUGH			
SPIT			
PURULENT SPIT			
WHEEZE			
CHEST PAIN			
BREATHLESSNESS			
NASAL SYMPTOMS			
OTHER (please specify)			

If symptom not mentioned by patient or by you - please leave blank

2. EXAMINATION

	Tick if exam-ined ✓	FINDINGS
CHEST		
THROAT		
GLANDS		
NOSE		
SINUSES		
EARS		

FEBRILE ON CLINICAL GROUNDS YES ☐ NO ☐

IF TEMPERATURE TAKEN, please indicate reading: ....°.

OTHER SIGNS (e.g. Breathlessness):

....

....

....

....

3. GENERAL

SELF MEDICATION FOR THIS ILLNESS	
ANY OTHER FEATURES INFLUENCING CURRENT TREATMENT (e.g. asthmatic chronic bronchitic)	

FOLLOW-UP: DEFINITELY ARRANGED ☐ ONLY IF PROGRESS UNSATISFACTORY ☐ (Please tick)

PLEASE STATE: Any Laboratory tests or X-Rays requested:

4. TREATMENT

4. TREATMENT	Nature of Advice (Please specify Drugs, e.g. Penicillin/Benylin, but NOT dosage)
BED REST	
STAY OFF WORK/SCHOOL	
STEAM INHALATION	
NASAL DROPS	
COUGH MIXTURE	
ANTIBIOTIC	
OTHER TREATMENT e.g. Aspirin, Paracetamol &c.	

5. SUMMARY

AGE OF PATIENT:........ SEX: ....

SEEN: AT HOME ☐ IN SURGERY ☐ (Please tick)

OCCUPATION (of Parent, if child): ....

Date of Consultation: ....

DIAGNOSIS: ....

proved that, with practice, completion of the form took well under one minute. The decision to put all the information on one side of the sheet followed a pilot run of a two-page form in one practice; the doctors reported that the document was unwieldy in that form and would have to be modified if they were going to take part in the study!

The second opening for criticism was the decision to select the doctors in the way described. Having decided against sampling from all British general practitioners because I felt that all prospective participants should be given the opportunity to discuss the project with me face-to-face, I was bound eventually to have to make generalisations from results collected from a selected sub-group of general practitioners. It seemed logical, therefore, to approach the sub-group of doctors which I felt would be most likely to help, namely doctors I know and doctors who had already shown an interest in the teaching side of general practice. In the end, the 63 doctors who agreed to help represented a sizeable proportion (25 per cent) of all the doctors in our then Executive Council area and, being 97 per cent of those doctors approached, could fairly be said to reflect a reasonable even if restricted spectrum of general practice opinion.

The third problem was the possibility that bias would be introduced by allowing doctors a measure of freedom to select consultations for inclusion in the study. Although I believed that my hypothesis was true for most respiratory illnesses and most general practitioners, I knew that heavy winter workload would make collection of detailed information on all respiratory consultations too demanding. For no particularly sound reason I felt confident that the degree of case selection I was proposing to allow would not greatly distort the spectrum of respiratory illness normally presented to general practitioners and that the flexible guidelines would result in a higher number of forms being completed.

The study took place from November and potential helpers were approached by letter and then by visit in early autumn. Before each month's recording was due, new forms were sent to each participant together with a progress report on the previous month's response for the complete project. Doctors from whom no response had been received were approached either by phone or letter to see if problems had arisen.

Two further points are worth emphasising. The first was the frustration at not receiving financial support from official state funds. Because the process of grant scrutiny is highly confidential no discussion of this failure to gain support can be presented here; suffice it to say that an opportunity to defend the application at an interview would have left a feeling that at least applicant and judges were fully aware of each others' aims and problems. The second difficulty was deciding how much of the aims of the study should be made known to the doctors being asked to help. I explained my belief that decisions to use antibiotics were probably related more closely to symptom/sign complexes than was often realised and that I wished to examine antibiotic use starting from this assumption. Perhaps this underplayed my full intentions; but it avoided leading the form of response by expanding on my view of the low value of many of the diagnostic labels routinely used in general practice.

Once again I was grateful for a mixture of good luck and massive support from my colleagues. A further influenza outbreak produced a January peak in illness which was reflected in a peak of forms returned, and the eventual total of 7,515 forms available for analysis gave every reason to suggest that respiratory illness had been fairly represented by the study as designed. (The main findings of the study are described on page 157.)

Project Three: 'Co-trimoxazole and Streptococcal Tonsillitis' (continued from page 55)

This study had clear aims, namely to 'compare the efficacy of high dose co-trimoxazole and oral penicillin V in the treatment of Group A beta-haemolytic streptococcal throat infections'. This project was the only one of the six presented in this chapter for which a formal protocol was written and it is ironic that the study should also have been the least successful. The main features of the design of the study – agreed between myself, a bacteriologist and the pharmaceutical company who initiated the idea – were as follows:

NUMERATOR	outcome to be measured (i) subjectively using patients' self-assessments of progress and side effects much as described in project one; (ii) objectively – the presence or absence of group A streptococci at one and four weeks, using throat swabs.
DENOMINATOR	patients presenting with acute throat infections, either sex, six years of age or over were eligible (*all* did not have to be entered). A number of exclusions were listed. Patients with positive throat swabs at first consultation to be

followed up at one and four weeks; those with negative swabs were not seen again unless clinically required. Doctors who were invited to take part were selected from a number known to swab throats routinely as part of their normal clinical practice.

TYPE OF STUDY — this study was a clinical trial, with the doctor (and patient) aware of the drug being taken. Commercially available preparations of co-trimoxazole and penicillin V were used. The treatment was to be allocated according to a randomisation chart.

METHOD OF COLLECTING INFORMATION — base-line, clinical and personal information was recorded on one half of a tear-off card which was then posted to myself as co-ordinator. The patient recorded progress on the other half for 14 days and then posted the card. Bacteriology reports were duplicated for routine and research use. Patient identity was retained by the general practitioner, and all documents labelled only with trial code number.

SIZE OF STUDY — the pharmaceutical company's statistician concluded that 100 patients with group A streptococci were required; we estimated that 20 doctors could recruit 20 patients each, over six months, to gain the necessary number of 'positives'.

ETHICS — at the time of starting the study no objections to the design or concept were raised; each general practitioner accepted that the final decision to include or exclude the patient was his. Important difficulties which arose later are discussed below.

FUNDING — by the pharmaceutical company; funds available included a modest item of service payment to the doctor for each patient recruited.

ORGANISATION — see below.

Three teaching practices who routinely swab their patients with sore throats were approached and, including three trainees, 15 doctors agreed to help. It was agreed that for adults the penicillin course would be 250 mg four times daily for seven days and that the course of co-trimoxazole would be three tablets twice daily for seven days. The study was intended to start on 1 November, but due to printing delays – not of our making – the working documents were not available until the last days of November. As a result, the recruitment of patients started – or failed to start – during the pre-Christmas period, several early cards were 'lost' in the Christmas mail and a general feeling of anti-climax was unavoidable. 'Spotted' tonsils proved much less common than any of the participants had expected (another lesson to be re-learned) and the inevitable preponderance of negative over positive swabs further reduced enthusiasm.

The main difficulty, however, arose from the development of itchy rashes in two of the first three co-trimoxazole takers, one on the sixth day of treatment and one on the day after completing treatment. An awkward ethical decision was unavoidable; were the rashes a chance coincidence or a significant result of high dose co-trimoxazole? The problem of continuing to use a second choice therapy of unproven clinical worth and now questionable safety had to be measured against the importance of 'proving' rather than merely suspecting a relationship between rash and treatment. Independent ethical advice was taken from three professional sources and all agreed the trial ought to be continued; it was, but doctors in the two practices in whom the patients with rashes had presented now started selecting patients for inclusion and exclusion depending on their knowledge of the next treatment indicated on their randomisation schedule. Two of the doctors in the third practice recruited no patients at any stage; these doctors had also been low contributors in project two. Hope of contributions from this practice was eventually abandoned and five additional doctors recruited.

After the Christmas break, recruiting improved and numbers began to match expectations. Patient response (66 per cent) as measured by replies received was about average and though adequate was well short of that achieved in project one. Motivation was understandably lower in both the doctors and patients. For a month no further adverse effects were reported; a rash in a penicillin-taker early in February confirmed the wisdom of the decision to continue the study and all seemed well. It was, of course, several weeks before a check showed that only three of the first eight 'positive' patients had been re-swabbed as required by the protocol and even after building in a double-check for this crucial aspect of determining the numerator, eleven of the subsequent twenty-seven patients missed one or both of their follow-up swabs. Too few as well as too many requirements reduce compliance;

patients do not visit doctors readily for follow-up when well; any procedure involving writing forms inhibits support; someone else's research is never as interesting as one's own.

The next problem that arose was almost a relief in that it provided grounds for halting the study which, in any case, was not producing enough material to reach its target before the now imminent summer holidays. A further rash in a co-trimoxazole taker was associated with a worrying neutropenia, and almost simultaneously a reply from a further patient reported a fourth rash developing shortly after completing a course of co-trimoxazole. The trial was stopped and review of the material started. The late replies brought one further rash in each group – a five to two preponderance with some fifty takers in each group. When, however, the penicillin-takers' rashes were examined further it became clear that the doctor entering the two patients had in error consistently reversed her codes and the two penicillin rashes in fact belonged to the co-trimoxazole group. Suspicion was immediately aroused that a 'german measles' in an incorrectly coded penicillin taker now represented an eighth co-trimoxazole rash and appropriate serology confirmed the suspicion by ruling out any past rubella infection. This eight-nil finding represented an unfortunate, but none the less important, conclusion to a chapter of miscalculations by several people involved in this study. Above all, this account emphasises the weakness of research organised by too many people with differing motives and expectations. I, at least, am unlikely to become involved again in a clinical trial that is not based on a double-blind and properly randomised design, or to support, without very careful thought, projects about which I do not have unreserved enthusiasm. I only hope these lessons have not been learned at any patient's lasting expense.

Salutary though this experience had been thus far, yet more was to be learned of the possible pitfalls of research! (This tale is concluded on page 159.)

Project Four: 'The Prevention of Adverse Drug Reactions' (continued from page 58).

In this project it was hoped to demonstrate a reduction in the prescribing of certain drugs to patients on anticoagulants when their record cards were tagged with appropriate warning labels. The design of the project centred on the region's anticoagulant register which included the names of all patients discharged from hospital on anticoagulant therapy. 442 patients were identified and their general practitioners were asked by letter if they would be willing to assist in 'a short project to examine the drug therapy being prescribed (to them) in addition to anticoagulants'. 85 patients who were no longer on anticongulants, or who had died, or whose doctors did not reply were excluded and 357 patients became the trial population. The letter to the doctor asked him to complete a card listing all medication prescribed to his patient(s) during the previous two months. Because the interaction between warfarin and barbiturates was regarded as being of particular importance, the patients were then divided into one group of 12 who had received barbiturates during the two-month period surveyed and the remainder (345) who had not. Test and control samples were drawn by allocating alternate patients from each group (barbiturate prescribed recently or not) to test or control groups; once one patient from a practice or a health centre had been allocated to one sample, all other patients looked after in the same premises were allocated to the same sample to avoid the difference between samples becoming obvious to participating doctors or ancillary staff. The profile of the project was as follows:

NUMERATOR	(i) the prescribing of barbiturates; (ii) the prescribing of other drugs listed in Figure 6.2 on page 56 during the six months of the study.
DENOMINATOR	all patients on anticoagulant whose doctors had indicated willingness to provide information on concurrent prescribing; patients randomly allocated to test and control samples (test sample issued with warning labels and drug card; control sample issued with drug card only) after stratification according to whether barbiturates had been prescribed in the preceding two months or not.
TYPE OF STUDY	combined retrospective and prospective.
METHOD OF COLLECTING INFORMATION	(i) copy of information extracted from existing practice record; (ii) collection of new information on record card designed for project.
SIZE OF STUDY	use of all information/patients available in local region; period of study – six months (December–May).
ETHICS	confidentiality protected by use of numbers.

FUNDING	postal and printing costs were estimated at around £100; this sum was met from money remaining unused from a larger unrelated project.
ORGANISATION	as described.

Having identified a large enough group of patients to ensure a satisfactory descriptive study (the study was eventually presented as an evaluation of a drug interaction warning system) and decided on the method and time scale, few difficulties were anticipated and none arose (with the possible exception of one doctor who asked to be paid for providing information for research purposes). After six months the doctors were asked to check the completeness of the entries on the drug card and return it in a stamped addressed envelope for photocopying. All but 14 of the records were returned for analysis. (The results of this study are summarised on page 160.)

Project Five: **'Can Clinical Judgement Be Analysed?'** (continued from page 59)

However diffuse or controversial the thinking behind this project may have been the eventual question asked and the hypothesis proposed were both clear. The development of the question 'Can I demonstrate how "patient" factors influence the clinical decisions taken by general practitioners?' to the hypothesis 'that awareness of non-physical features in a consultation for physical illness (in this case the symptom of sore throat with the sign of localised redness) may influence in a measurable way the doctor's decision to prescribe a physical remedy (in this case an antibiotic)' was traced in Chapter 6 and the idea of experimenting with photographic techniques in the testing of the hypothesis introduced. The profile of the project developed as follows:

NUMERATOR	answers of YES or NO to the question 'Would you prescribe an antibiotic?' posed in relation to a series of illustrated case histories presented in booklet form (the histories varied from booklet to booklet only in details of psychosocial background; the illustrations and other clinical details were kept constant).
DENOMINATOR	one thousand doctors selected haphazardly from the medical directory and assumed to be general practitioners because of possession of

	the MRCGP/FRCGP diploma; doctors working in my own geographical area, in university departments or possibly not in active practice were excluded. The doctors selected were randomly allocated one of six different booklets each containing different combinations of the possible psychosocial background features as described below.
TYPE OF STUDY	prospective; using simulation of clinical problems.
METHOD OF COLLECTING INFORMATION	responses to questions asked in a booklet constructed for the purposes of the study.
SIZE OF STUDY	1,000 doctors – hoping for a 50 per cent response which would allow an easy but informative statistical analysis of the replies by hand.
ETHICS	no apparent ethical difficulties; the patients whose throats were photographed knew the material would be used for teaching and research purposes without their identities being disclosed.
FUNDING	the postal and stationery costs (£150) were met by a grant from a pharmaceutical company to which previous unpaid services had been given; the costs of the development of the technical aspects of the project were absorbed as a part of the University of Aberdeen's medical illustration service.
ORGANISATION	discussed below.

In its simplest form the idea was to prepare twelve clinical problems each with:

(i) the same clinical background (detailed in the preface to the booklet – Figure 10.5);
(ii) a reproduction of an inflamed throat special to that problem; and
(iii) one of a pair of alternative psychosocial background statements special to that problem.

Figure 10.5: Background Clinical Information Applicable to All Problems Presented in Booklet

UNLESS STATED TO THE CONTRARY:

All patients are being seen at the doctor's surgery in the middle of a winter week; respiratory illness though prevalent is not reaching epidemic proportions. The practice is a 4 man group practice serving a quarter of the local market town of 30 000 patients and rural areas in a ten mile radius from it.

All patients have presented with a complaint of *sore throat* of 24 hours duration partly helped by salicylates but having interfered with sleep the previous night. None of the patients is allergic to any drugs and none have significant past histories of illness of respiratory or other nature.

It should be assumed that patients are in contact with coryzal illness and although not currently suffering from typical symptoms of coryza are complaining of feeling generally unwell as if developing 'flu'. The chest and ear drums are normal; the patients are *not* fevered and have neither cough nor sputum; they are non-smokers. All have some small glands palpable in the tonsillar region; these are slightly tender on deep palpation.

You are asked to state **YES** or **NO** to the question
Would you prescribe an antibiotic ?
given: i) the information above
ii) the photograph of the throat as shown
iii) the additional information below each photograph.

Doctors vary widely in the frequency with which they prescribe antibiotics to patients with sore throats and I had to assume that if my population of 1,000 doctors was divided into two groups of 500, equal numbers in the two groups would elect to 'prescribe' an antibiotic for each of the pictures reproduced as in (ii) above. I had next to show that if one of the groups of 500 doctors was given a more emotive added psychological background history the prescribing rate would then differ between the two groups.

The first technical problem lay in using reproductions that looked too normal (for whom no one would prescribe no matter what the non-physical influences) or too abnormal (for whom nearly everyone would prescribe irrespective of non-physical influences). The second problem lay in the possibility that colour intensity would 'drift' during a large printing run, introducing bias to responses as a result. The first problem was tackled by photographing some sixty throats – mainly in one busy eight-doctor health centre – and selecting the most suitable pictures for further processing.

The sixteen chosen illustrations were then reproduced on four A4 sheets, each including four pictures. The second problem was tackled by incorporating in each of these pages of four pictures one 'control' picture in which the added psychological history was kept constant for the complete printing run despite changes being made halfway through the run to the psychosocial histories added to the other three pictures (Figure 10.6).

The cover of each booklet incorporated the introductory clinical notes and a tear-off reply card (using a business reply licence) including a space for the name and address of the replying doctor for use if he wished to receive a copy of the results. The central part of each booklet presented sixteen 'patients', twelve being included as test patients and four as colour controls. To allow for the necessary mixing of the types of psychosocial history when binding of the four sets of four pictures took place, the 'patients' were distributed amongst the printed A4 sheets as follows:

	Test Patients			Control Patients
SHEET 1	4	13	16	1
SHEET 2	2	3	14	15
SHEET 3	5	8	9	12
SHEET 4	7	10	11	6

500 copies of each sheet were printed with the 'neutral' psychosocial histories for the test patients; 500 copies with the 'provocative' psychosocial histories. Each booket was composed using two 'neutral' sheets and two 'provocative' sheets. Six combinations of sheets were thus possible all avoiding runs of one or other type of psychosocial history. The content of each booklet was

Figure 10.6: One Page of Reproductions Including Four Reproductions (psychosocial histories below patients 7, 10, 11 changed in middle of printing run but history below patient 6 held constant)

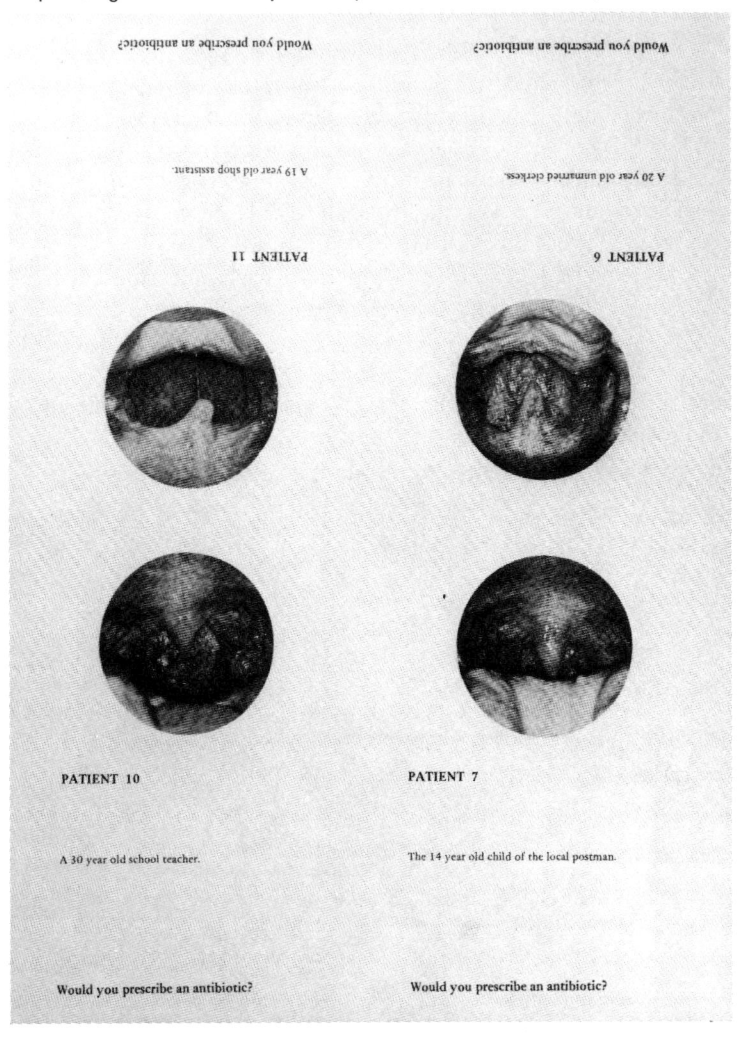

PATIENT 11

A 19 year old shop assistant.

Would you prescribe an antibiotic?

PATIENT 6

A 20 year old unmarried clerkess.

Would you prescribe an antibiotic?

PATIENT 10

A 30 year old school teacher.

Would you prescribe an antibiotic?

PATIENT 7

The 14 year old child of the local postman.

Would you prescribe an antibiotic?

indicated by a combination of circles on the edge of the reply card. The outside cover of the booklet, the facing of the reply card which opened out from the last page and the fully opened booklet are shown in Figure 10.7.

These design features have been described in detail to illustrate, not how complex research design is, but how logical and thus simple it becomes when potential difficulties are allowed for at the planning stage. Had this project not been carefully thought through at this juncture, the replies which were received (over 600) might have proved impossible to interpret. As it was the analysis and interpretation of the replies received proved remarkably straightforward.

The selection of doctors for circulation was haphazard rather than random and my sample could only claim to reflect all general

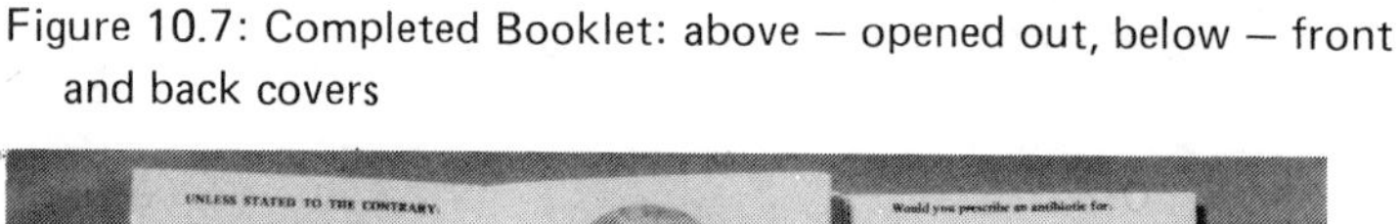
Figure 10.7: Completed Booklet: above — opened out, below — front and back covers

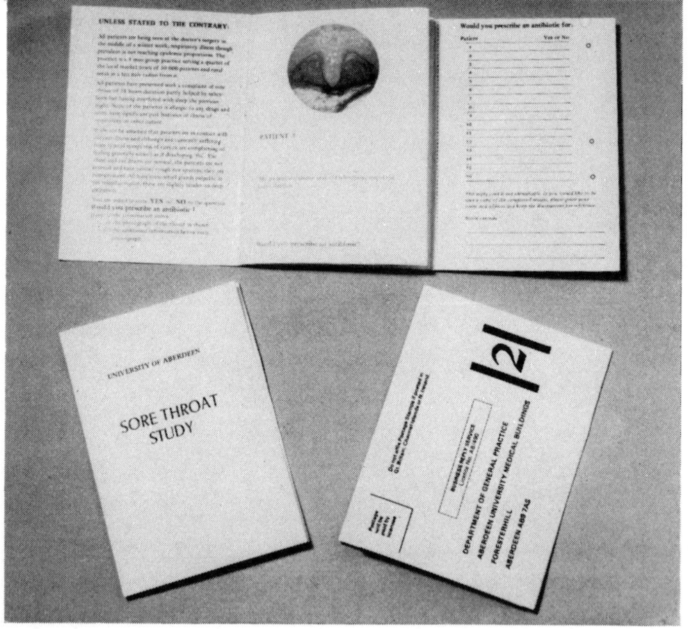

Figure 10.8: Covering Letter Posted with Booklet

UNIVERSITY OF ABERDEEN

PROFESSOR I. M. RICHARDSON
TEL. NO. 23423
Ext. 2516

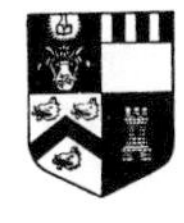

DEPARTMENT OF GENERAL PRACTICE
UNIVERSITY MEDICAL BUILDINGS
FORESTERHILL, ABERDEEN
AB9 2ZD

April 1976

Dear

Treatment of Sore Throats

Discussion of the indications for use of antibiotics in patients with sore throats has been confused by diagnostic terms (tonsillitis, pharyngitis) and descriptive terms (inflamed, injected) which mean different things to different doctors.

I am trying to get round this by using photographs of the throats of patients who have complained of this common symptom and adding relevant notes about their histories and circumstances.

In order to try to build a consensus view of appropriate general practice management for teaching purposes, I would appreciate knowing whether or not you would have prescribed antibiotics in the situations presented in this enclosed booklet. Please use the tear-off reply-paid card inside the back cover for your reply.

Your name is one of several hundred chosen randomly from doctors in the Medical Register with an MRCGP or FRCGP. The reply card is totally anonymous but if you wish to be sent a copy of the overall results please add your name and address to the reply card.

The success of the venture depends on a high reply rate. The booklet should not take much more than 5 minutes to complete; if you are willing to help please return the card as soon as possible. If more than one partner in your practice has received a booklet, please complete the card without comparing notes!

Thank you for helping.

Yours sincerely,

J.G.R. Howie

practitioners were it known that, for example, all general practitioners send entries to the Medical Directory, and that those general practitioners who are holders of the MRCGP/FRCGP are no different from those who are not (a subject for a research project at another time!). My hypothesis did not require me to sample *all* general practitioners, and this issue did not seem crucial. What was important was to waste as few circulars as possible.

My belief in the importance of presenting material as attractively and personally as possible resulted in the printing of the letter shown in Figure 10.8. This letter was headed, dated and signed by hand for all the doctors being asked to help and put in envelopes which again I addressed personally by hand. The letter told enough about the aims of the project to explain why help was being asked, but neither too much, which might have influenced replies, nor too little, which might have misled. Doctors replying could choose anonymity or not as they wished.

The difficulties involved in reproducing the photographs cannot be done justice to here. Several practice runs had to be discarded and even then much of the final production run was rejected for technical reasons. Here the value of the 'technical' control proved itself and analyses of replies to the 'control' problems suggested that a satisfactory level of technical consistency had eventually been achieved. The immense enthusiasm of my colleagues in this field was an absolute requirement for the success of this venture and a clear acknowledgement of the importance of their help is an appropriate way to finish this description of the methods used for this project. (The main conclusions of this study are presented on page 161.)

Project Six: 'Prescribing to Save Work' (continued from page 61)

Projects can be preceded by an exploratory feasibility study to see if an apparently interesting idea can be studied using a particular technique. During this often brief exercise, weaknesses of a proposed method can be identified, the likely quantity of available material gauged and potentially interesting alternative or future questions recognised. Although this particular study is presented last, its simple conception and design probably reflect most closely the approach that a doctor attempting research for the first time might use.

The project was designed to assess the progress of patients with acute respiratory illness, who had been seen by various doctors who had different antibiotic prescribing policies, but were all working in the same practice. Outcome was to be regarded as unsatisfactory if patients consulted again within two weeks of their original consultation and

(i) received an antibiotic when one had not been prescribed initially – or
(ii) received a change of antibiotic after an antibiotic had been prescribed initially.

The profile of the project was as follows:

NUMERATOR	all apparently new respiratory consultations which had been recorded between 1970 and 1976 inclusive divided into those where (i) a further consultation took place within two weeks and either an antibiotic was prescribed after having not been prescribed initially or a prescription for a second and different antibiotic was given and (ii) no change in antibiotic prescribing policy took place within two weeks of the original consultation.
DENOMINATOR	three groups of patients who had been registered with the practice throughout their lives were studied: (i) all those born in 1970; (ii) all those born in 1960 and (iii) all those born in 1950 or 1951. Note was made of the doctor carrying out each consultation studied.
TYPE OF STUDY	retrospective study of practice records.
METHOD OF COLLECTING INFORMATION	handwritten lists after study of individual record envelopes; the patients identified from the practice age-sex register.
SIZE OF STUDY	the records were examined for the period from 1970 to 1976 inclusive. 50 patients were identified in the first age-group described above, and 60 and 43 in the second and third age-groups.
ETHICS	confidentiality of information had to be protected.
FUNDING	no costs incurred.
ORGANISATION	as described.

The organisation of the study was straightforward and the main problem for the doctor undertaking the work was being able to recognise and read the handwriting of the doctors who had made the entries in the records. The issue of the accuracy and completeness of the records was, of course, an important one and is discussed later. It is worth repeating that the design of this project was felt to be adequate for no more than a cautious descriptive study with limited aims and that, at this stage, no hypothesis was under test. (The findings from this study are presented on page 163.)

The better of these six projects share common characteristics which should be re-emphasised.

The numerator should be simple and objective – a decision to prescribe or not prescribe a drug, to do or not to do an investigation, to refer or not to refer. The denominator or population being studied should be defined in advance of the study in as much detail as possible and after careful thought of what sub-groups might be analysed separately at a later stage. The population studied should be one which is likely to be easily available for study and preferably one that is likely to be co-operative. New information is usually a sounder basis for research than information collected for some other purpose, provided that the information can be collected without introducing bias on the part of the observer (often the doctor) or the subject (often the patient). The risks of collecting either too little or too much information can be reduced by having a clear statement of aims or a hypothesis before planning begins. Studies where plenty of time is taken before a final design is agreed are preferable to those where planning is rushed and studies where participants share a high level of interest are more likely to succeed than those where motivation is uneven or absent. Expensive projects have no necessary merit over inexpensive projects. And the credentials of ethically acceptable research should include sound design and positively exclude unsound design!

PART THREE

LOOKING AT RESULTS

11 ANALYSING RESULTS

Information collected has now to be grouped into categories (classified) which are then allocated numbers to simplify their analysis (coded). These code numbers may then be transferred to cards or similar material (data preparation) for analysis by sorting machines, or computers, or even by hand (data handling). This chapter covers these activities.

A number of general points should be appreciated before analysis starts.

1. Even efficient analysis of results may take many months to complete. It is common for interest to flag, particularly when problems seem to be emerging faster than answers. Be reassured that this is a common experience and press on as quickly as possible. The longer difficulties are shelved the more likely it is that they will never be tackled and that the research will be left unfinished.
2. If the research has been poorly conceived, carelessly designed, or inconsistently carried out these basic defects cannot now be rectified.
3. *No methods of analysis and no statistical procedures can convert poor-quality information into good-quality results.*
4. The kinds of analyses which will be necessary will depend in part on what tests or procedures will be required for statistical interpretation of the results. Further discussions with a statistician are advisable. If this is not done analyses may have to be duplicated at a later stage, tabulations reconstructed and even classifications re-ordered.
5. Having more information, rather than less information, available does not necessarily make analysis and interpretation of research easier. The use of a computer does not by itself guarantee that results will be produced faster and more efficiently than when simpler methods are used.

Classification

Ideal classes or categories are those which are objective and discrete and thus both include all information which is relevant and exclude all which is not. Sex, for instance, is easily classified and age is easily classified in chronological terms, but not so easily in biological terms. Response to treatment may be readily classified at a crude level (death or survival) but is often extremely difficult to classify at the finer levels of quality of survival. Attitudes and opinions may be particularly difficult to classify, especially when respondents are left free to state their own responses. However, the restriction of responses which results from designing 'closed' as against 'open' questionnaires or research records, although making classification technically easier, may introduce spurious accuracy.

A question about the working of an appointment system might be framed thus:

> 'Are you satisfied with the present arrangements for making appointments?' ....

or thus:

> 'Please indicate which statement most closely represents your view of our present arrangements for making appointments.'
>
> 1. ALWAYS SATISFACTORY
> 2. USUALLY SATISFACTORY
> 3. OFTEN SATISFACTORY
> 4. OFTEN UNSATISFACTORY
> 5. USUALLY UNSATISFACTORY
> 6. ALWAYS UNSATISFACTORY

Faced with the first opportunity to voice particular grievances a respondent might answer: 'Works alright when you speak to the older receptionist.' The respondent might pick any boxes from 2 to 5 when given option two, none of the choices in which fully reflect his or her point of view. (One way out of this difficulty is to have an 'open' option in an otherwise 'closed' question; in the above example a final box: OTHER (PLEASE DESCRIBE) might be left available for respondents who did not feel the other choices adequate.)

Inaccuracy in classification may also be produced when different observers classify similar responses in different ways, when one observer classifies similar material inconsistently and when replies are forced into available categories for reasons of convenience rather than logic. Clearly much thought has to be given to the intellectual integrity of whatever system of classification of material is to be used, because once classes have been defined and material allocated to them the rest of the chain of events involved in analysis and interpretation can follow almost automatically.

Several systems of classification have evolved over many years and give results which are sufficiently consistent and reproducible for many purposes. One of the better examples is the Registrar General's *Classification of Occupations* (1970); occupation is classified differently according to whether employment status, economic position or social or socio-economic status is being considered. The commonly used social class groupings are based on this classification and detailed working instructions are published with it. The usefulness of this and any other system depends on the accuracy and completeness of the information available; terms such as, for instance, 'engineer' are too vague to classify accurately and, in addition, the information on occupation on record envelopes is all too often out of date.

A number of systems of classifying diseases or symptoms are available. The most commonly used is the ICD (*International Classification of Diseases*, 1978) which is presented in two complementary volumes and is available in all medical libraries. The RCGP modification of the ICD (known as the *College Classification*, 1963) contains fewer categories and makes allowance for the range of illnesses as seen in general practice, and the way they present. The ICHPPC (*An International Classification of the Health Problems of Primary Care*, 1976) represents an attempt to cover both psychosocial and clinical morbidity, but its role may have been overtaken by the inclusion in the ninth edition of the ICD of specific categories for domestic and psychosocial problems. As well as depending on the availability of good-quality information, the usefulness of these classifications depends on uniform interpretation of information by those undertaking the classification.

Before classification of results is started, the details of the design of the classification to be used should be written down. Clear instructions should be included on how to deal with categories such as 'no reply', 'no return' and 'don't know'. Often other difficulties may be forestalled by a preliminary scanning of the replies or results of a study. The list of instructions on how to operate the classification will usually be added to as further information is dealt with and sometimes the 'ifs' and 'buts' become so numerous that a basic change in the system has to be made and the process re-started. Galling though this is, it is better faced early in the analysis of a study than after everything has been classified, coded and analysed. Some of the material should be re-classified by the original observer and also by a second observer to check the consistency of both the system and its operators. Finally, I strongly advise any research worker to undertake at least part of this work personally, as this often helps the recognition of associations or trends in the findings which might otherwise be missed. Problems in the use of the classification can also be identified and dealt with early and efficiently.

Coding

Coding is simply the allocation of a different symbol (usually a number) to each category defined during classification of the material in the research record. As it is customary to allocate code numbers direct from raw information it may seem pedantic to draw a distinction between classification and coding. Indeed, what has already been said about classification also applies to coding. However, one important change takes place during coding, and this is the conversion either of *verbal* information to *numerical* information, or of one type of numerical information to a different type.

(i) Verbal information may be allocated a number such as 789.2 (abdominal pain in the ICD) which is different from another, for example, 786.2 (cough in the ICD) without the numbers indicating any relationship between the qualities. In addition, none or several of a range of qualities may be present, and the range of code numbers must allow for this. For example, responses to a question on 'presenting symptoms' might be coded as follows:

CODE	DESCRIPTION
1	cough
2	sore throat
3	sore ear
4	abdominal pain
5	other symptoms
6	no entry
7	cough + sore throat
8	cough + sore ear. . .
9	. . .and so on

The only arithmetical procedure possible during analysis of such codings is the demonstration of the distribution of information between the categories chosen.

(ii) Alternatively, verbal information may indicate the presence of qualities which may be regarded as 'better or worse' or 'more or less' and can be ranked. Code number 1 might, for example, be more desirable (cure) than number 2 (improved) which in turn would be better than 3 and 4 (unchanged or worse). Number 5 (deceased) would be less desirable still. Although the categories are separated by a constant numerical interval, an equal step numerically does not necessarily imply an equal step clinically (1 to 2, compared with 4 to 5) and the ways in which the data can be used arithmetically may again be restricted. When a ranking scale is used each record can, of course, only be placed in one category and the problems of coding permutations of, for example, multiple diagnoses or multiple drug therapies are avoided.

(iii) When numerical values are classified and converted to code the problems are obvious. Clearly a range of code numbers identical, for example, to age by decade permits a variety of arithmetical deductions to be made from their subsequent analyses. If, however, the classification of age selected was as follows:

CODE	DESCRIPTION
1	first year of life
2. . .	second year of life. . .
. . .6	. . .sixth year of life
7	seven to nine years
8	ten to nineteen years
9	twenty or over
0	no entry

a different range of arithmetical manoeuvres would be possible after analysis of the results.

In the past information was normally transcribed to punch cards with 80 columns of figures, each column offering the range of codes 0–9 inclusive together with X and Y. Classifications including no more than twelve possibilities per item were thus desirable as those with more required more complex sorting of the punch cards. The advent of modern methods of data processing has eased this restriction, but increasing the possible range of code numbers relating to one item can encourage the use of excessively long lists of sub-categories. Some of these may be used so seldom during analysis that in the end aggregation of categories has to be undertaken to provide figures large enough to interpret statistically.

Data Preparation and Handling

The methods available for analysing information range from simple hand sorting of annotated cards or other records, through hand sorting of cards prepared with edge punching, to the machine sorting of cards with coded information punched centrally. The computer, which works from data stored on magnetic tape, is an extension of the principle of the centre-punch record.

Research records where coded numbers are made to stand out prominently by, for example, the use of coloured ink may be suitable for analysis as they stand. Hand sorting of records is usually possible when the total number of records is small, the number of variables being studied small, or the possible number of sub-divisions of each item limited. Defining the limits of what can be tackled this way is difficult; provided analyses are done tidily and methodically and the results noted carefully, it should be possible to handle several hundred records without undue difficulty. Although hand analysis can be time consuming it is not prohibitively so and the researcher depends on no one for the use of time or machines, has no queues to join and no emergencies to make way for. Doing everything personally allows recognition of sequences of results and correlations which might easily be missed when machine sorting is undertaken by a research clerk. Card rather than paper records should be used as paper handles less well than card and deteriorates quicker.

The edge-punch research record also saves the need for machines and requires only a punching tool and knitting needle. This card carries information on its outer rims with holes punched to correspond to the selected codes. Single items may be recognised as present or absent by punching or not punching the appropriate position on the card edge. Further detail can be obtained by taking four holes to indicate one attribute and regarding them as of code value 1, 2, 4 and 7 respectively. By punching various combinations of these four holes any value for the attribute (age, diagnosis, length of symptoms, for example) from 1 to 14 can be recorded. An example of what is commonly known as a cope-chat card (Copeland-Chatterson) is shown in Figure 11.1.

This card has over 100 holes round its four edges and additional information can be entered on the back and front of the record. The cards and punching tool are available commercially and even if modestly expensive are much cheaper than buying computer time![1] It is, of course, possible to make one's own simple punch card using a postcard, or some other record such as an age-sex register card. Heavy pencil or

Figure 11.1: A Cope-Chat (Edge-punch) Card

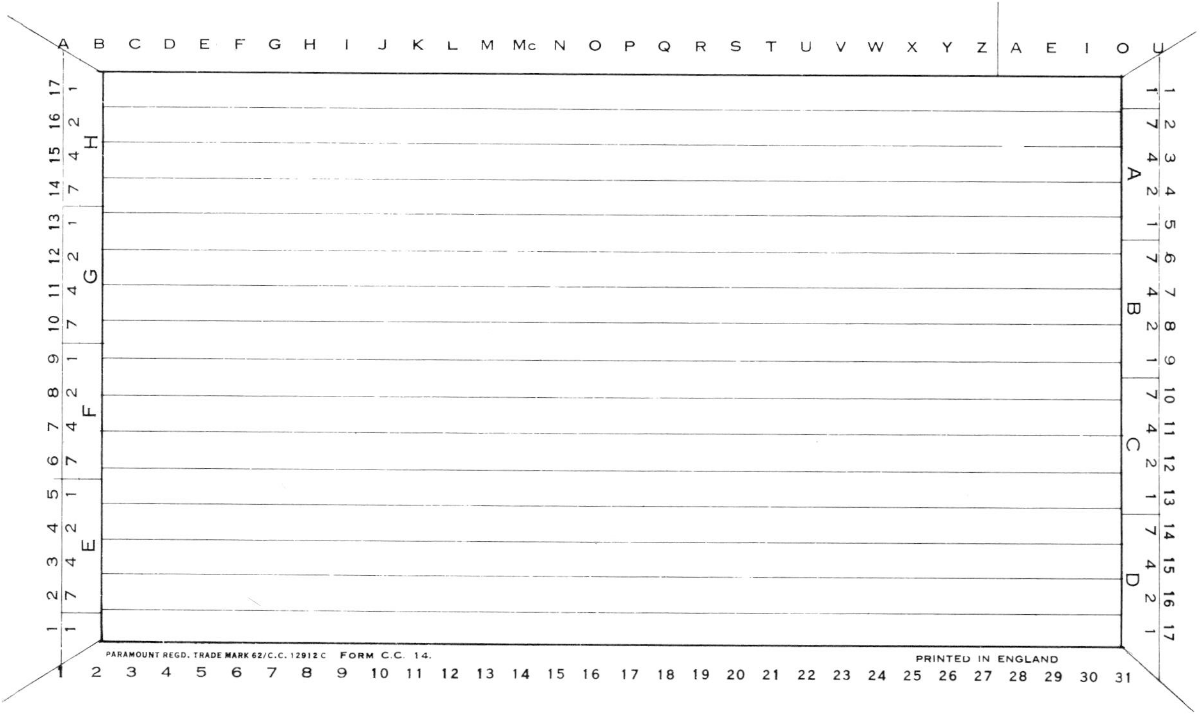

Figure 11.2: A Centre-punch Record Card

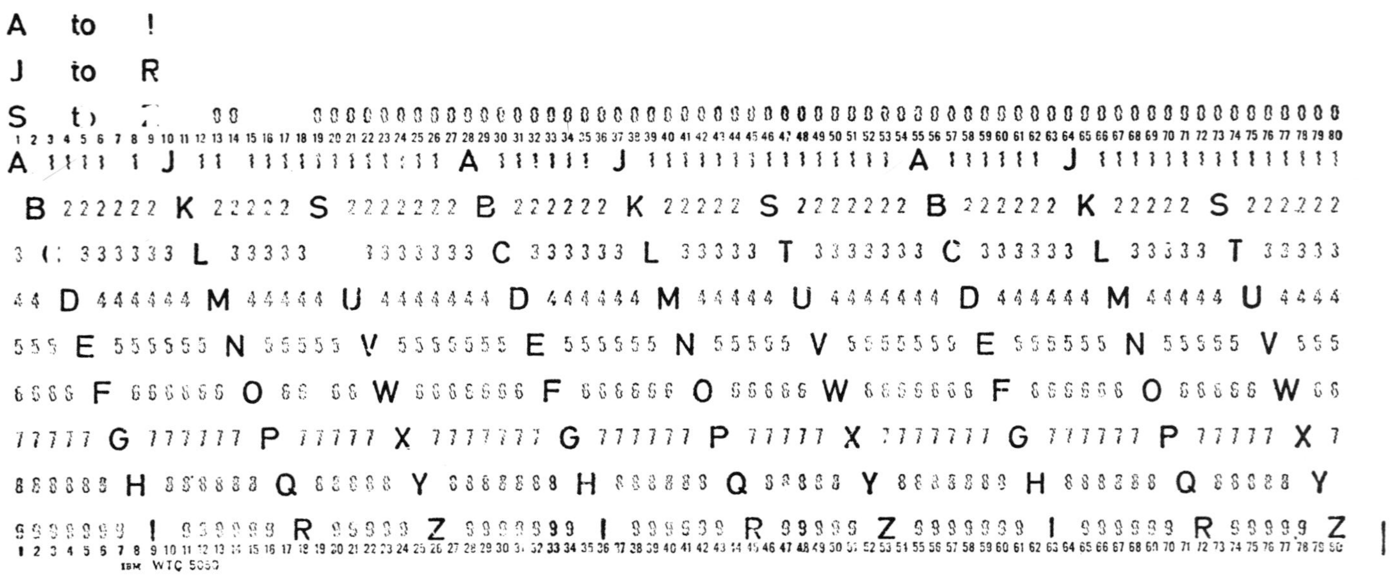

A to I

J to R

S to Z

```
              0 0     0 0 0 0 0 0 0 0 0 0 0 0 0 0 0 0 0 0 0 0 0 0 0 0 0 0 0 0 0 0 0 0 0 0 0 0 0 0 0 0 0 0 0 0 0 0 0 0 0 0 0 0 0 0 0 0 0 0 0 0
1 2 3 4 5 6 7 8 9 10 11 12 13 14 15 16 17 18 19 20 21 22 23 24 25 26 27 28 29 30 31 32 33 34 35 36 37 38 39 40 41 42 43 44 45 46 47 48 49 50 51 52 53 54 55 56 57 58 59 60 61 62 63 64 65 66 67 68 69 70 71 72 73 74 75 76 77 78 79 80
A 1 1 1 1   1 J 1 1   1 1 1 1 1 1 1 1 1 1 1 1 1 1 A 1 1 1 1 1 1   J 1 1 1 1 1 1 1 1 1 1 1 1 1 1 1 1 A 1 1 1 1 1 1   J 1 1 1 1 1 1 1 1 1 1 1 1 1 1 1 1
 B 2 2 2 2 2 2 K 2 2 2 2 2 S 2 2 2 2 2 2 2 B 2 2 2 2 2 2 K 2 2 2 2 2 S 2 2 2 2 2 2 2 B 2 2 2 2 2 2 K 2 2 2 2 2 S 2 2 2 2 2 2
3     3 3 3 3 3 3 L 3 3 3 3 3       3 3 3 3 3 3 3 C 3 3 3 3 3 3 L 3 3 3 3 3 T 3 3 3 3 3 3 3 C 3 3 3 3 3 3 L 3 3 3 3 3 T 3 3 3 3 3
4 4 D 4 4 4 4 4 4 M 4 4 4 4 4 U 4 4 4 4 4 4 4 D 4 4 4 4 4 4 M 4 4 4 4 4 U 4 4 4 4 4 4 4 D 4 4 4 4 4 4 M 4 4 4 4 4 U 4 4 4 4
5 5 5 E 5 5 5 5 5 5 N 5 5 5 5 5 V 5 5 5 5 5 5 5 E 5 5 5 5 5 5 N 5 5 5 5 5 V 5 5 5 5 5 5 5 E 5 5 5 5 5 5 N 5 5 5 5 5 V 5 5 5
6 6 6 6 F 6 6 6 6 6 6 O 6 6   6 6 W 6 6 6 6 6 6 6 F 6 6 6 6 6 6 O 6 6 6 6 6 W 6 6 6 6 6 6 6 F 6 6 6 6 6 6 O 6 6 6 6 6 W 6 6
7 7 7 7 7 G 7 7 7 7 7 7 P 7 7 7 7 7 X 7 7 7 7 7 7 7 G 7 7 7 7 7 7 P 7 7 7 7 7 X 7 7 7 7 7 7 7 G 7 7 7 7 7 7 P 7 7 7 7 7 X 7
8 8 8 8 8 8 H 8 8 8 8 8 8 Q 8 8 8 8 8 Y 8 8 8 8 8 8 8 H 8 8 8 8 8 8 Q 8 8 8 8 8 Y 8 8 8 8 8 8 8 H 8 8 8 8 8 8 Q 8 8 8 8 8 Y
9 9 9 9 9 9 9 I 9 9 9 9 9 9 R 9 9 9 9 9 Z 9 9 9 9 9 9 9 I 9 9 9 9 9 9 R 9 9 9 9 9 Z 9 9 9 9 9 9 9 I 9 9 9 9 9 9 R 9 9 9 9 9 Z
1 2 3 4 5 6 7 8 9 10 11 12 13 14 15 16 17 18 19 20 21 22 23 24 25 26 27 28 29 30 31 32 33 34 35 36 37 38 39 40 41 42 43 44 45 46 47 48 49 50 51 52 53 54 55 56 57 58 59 60 61 62 63 64 65 66 67 68 69 70 71 72 73 74 75 76 77 78 79 80
      IBM WTC 5050
```

pen markings at the card edge will also stand out when a pack of records are stacked together for sorting. The proper edge-punch card is sorted using a knitting needle; home-made cards may require a little more ingenuity.

The centre-punch card requires more elaborate machinery for both preparation and sorting. One of its advantages is that it can carry more information than an edge-punch card. An example of a centre-punch card is shown in Figure 11.2. This card (the Hollerith card) has to be punched on one machine and sorted on another which may, in addition, count while sorting. The cards have 80 columns of figures, each column offering a choice of twelve positions for punching. Professional punch-card operators can prepare as many as 200 cards in an hour. The cards deteriorate if not stored properly (tightly packed in a cool, dry store) and can only be sorted a limited number of times (perhaps 100 to 200), before the edges become machine worn and unusable. The sorting machine takes nearly ten minutes to sort 500 cards for one item of information, so analyses involving other than simple breakdowns and correlations become quite time consuming. Punch cards prepared for a Hollerith sorter can in turn provide the raw material for transfer to magnetic tape for computer analysis and information on magnetic tape can be returned to punch cards for storage. Although the Hollerith card is the best known example of a centre-punch card, some interest has focused recently on the Jolley feature card as a means of storing information on practice morbidity and patient characteristics. This method also requires machine punching and although simple analyses can be done by hand, special equipment is again required for more complex analyses.[2]

When information is presented for analysis it should be marshalled in a neat and clear manner already checked for accuracy. Many data-processing centres will request that 'raw' data is presented on forms designed to their own requirements and generally data processors will prefer to operate from horizontal lines of code rather than vertical lines. When the material has been punched, the accuracy of the punching is usually confirmed by a checking process; but the accuracy of the *initial* material can only be checked to a limited extent by screening for 'impossible' codes (for example, if 'sex' is recorded as 0-male, 1-female, 2-not recorded, then any entries of three or higher would be rejected: no check on the accuracy or otherwise of entries within the range of 0-2 can, of course, be made).

The processing of information by computer has been one of the most important research developments in recent years, and present indications are that analysis of results using the Hollerith card and counter-sorter will become a chapter in history within a few years. The computer can analyse enormous quantities of data in complex ways with great speed and great accuracy (human errors excepted!). Its advantages in the analysis of large scale studies are significant. The drawbacks lie in the risks of machine breakdown, having to wait for access or to make way for 'emergencies', having to meet expenses if realistic fees are charged and often the need to adapt information to fit with the capabilities of available 'programmes' for analysis of data. It is not widely appreciated how time consuming the writing and checking of a new programme can be and how scarce are those with the ability to do this task. There is little chance of a single-handed research worker having a programme prepared specially for his needs, but the SPSS (Statistical Programme for the Social Sciences) has been particularly designed to meet the needs of research of the type likely to be undertaken in general practice. Yet again, it has to be stressed that the use of a computer cannot compensate for poor planning of research and that the possibility of access to one of these remarkable machines should not be seen as an excuse for the unselective collection of a mass of haphazard information.

Analysis. When results are being analysed by hand methods, or using a counter-sorter, it often helps to reduce the number of cards being handled at any one time by separating cards or records into those related, for example, to male and female patients, or test and control patients, or various age groups of patients. Subsequent analysis can then concentrate on breaking these more manageable quantities into whatever smaller categories seem of interest. On the other hand, particularly when computers are being used, it may be a better use of time to start by breaking information into small categories and then add these together for further examination: for instance, totals of consultations broken down by age of patient, day of week, and whether carried out at home or in the surgery, can be added in various ways from a single initial analysis. With these two differing approaches different risks are taken. If the first approach is taken interesting findings may be overlooked because of excessive crudeness of the breakdown; if, in contrast, over-elaborate analyses are attempted the resulting small allocations to individual categories may lead to interesting trends being missed. Once again, it is easier to decide the course to take if the aims of the study are clear in advance of the analysis starting.

When a large amount of information is available it is always tempting to try to correlate everything with everything else. In most studies the design will have concentrated on one or a few central pieces of information and these will probably be of better quality than others collected as a secondary part of the study. Analyses involving information which is of uncertain reliability may be of use in providing leads for further studies; but responsibility and judgement have to be used in deciding at what point the confidence that can be placed in apparent associations falls below the known quality of the recorded information.

Analyses made should always be neatly and clearly recorded and totals and sub-totals cross-checked for accuracy as and when possible. *Every* table or breakdown should be informatively labelled so that checks, additions or subtractions can be made if required. Some people have a great ability to look at tables or figures and detect trends or suggest further analyses which others may have missed or misinterpreted. Before regarding analysis as complete it is worth exploring this possibility with a friend or colleague who has some experience in research and possibly knows of the thinking behind the project concerned.

Do not throw away any of the records you have used for your research at this stage. Indeed these should probably be kept for several years after the results have been finalised and published so that questions on the work can be answered, or further analyses made, if required.

Notes

1. Information on Cope-Chat cards from Copeland-Chatterson Co. Ltd, 17 Waterloo Place, London SW1Y 4AR.
2. Information on the Jolley feature card system from Information Systems &Services Ltd, Westbourne Street, High Wycombe, Bucks.

References

Classification of Occupations, Office of Population Censuses and Surveys (HMSO, London, 1970).
College of General Practitioners, 'A Classification of Disease', *Journal of the College of General Practitioners*, 6 (1963), pp.204-16.
International Classification of Diseases (World Health Organisation, Geneva, 1978).
'An International Classification of the Health Problems of Primary Care', *Journal of the Royal College of General Practitioners,* Occasional Paper no.1 (1976).

12 INTERPRETING RESULTS

It is surprising that doctors, despite an essentially scientific training, should so often lack confidence in their ability to interpret research findings. This applies not only to the analysis of current research studies but also to work published in the medical press, presented at scientific meetings, or used to promote pharmaceutical products.

If this lack of confidence is surprising, its origins are probably reasonably easy to identify. Medical journals have tended to over-emphasise the importance of tests of statistical significance in deciding what to publish and educators (in the broadest and often amateur sense) have tended to base their messages on an often uncritical acceptance of these statistical findings. Undue concentration on statistics and statistical significance, which few doctors understand well enough to discuss let alone debate, has diverted attention from the other two major issues which must also be satisfied before any interpretation of findings can be accepted as reasonable:

was the information submitted to the tests of statistical significance of adequate quality?
are the findings and conclusions being presented of clinical importance?

General practitioners have developed the ability to make intuitive assessments of the relevance to themselves and their patients of much of what is described as 'research'. It is unfortunate that they do not often enough follow these judgements by identifying the precise weaknesses of the studies concerned and making their views known.

In this chapter I want to discuss interpretation of results under the three headings of 'Validity and Reliability', 'Statistical Significance' and 'Clinical Significance'. I will suggest first that no tests of statistical significance should be applied to material the validity and reliability of which has not been thoughtfully assessed, and secondly that the discussion of clinical significance should be given greater attention in the presentation of results than is often the case at present.

Validity and Reliability

The concepts of validity and reliability of research methods were introduced and discussed when the design of research was considered earlier in the book (page 75) A method is 'valid' when it measures what it sets out to measure with acceptable accuracy. What will be regarded as an acceptable level of accuracy may vary according to the aims of different projects. A method is 'reliable' when it produces consistent results and again an acceptable level of reliability has to be decided for a given method and a given study. Validity and reliability of method and information add together to equal the 'quality' of what is available for analysis and interpretation.

Validity of a method is assessed by comparing results produced using the method with those produced using other standard methods. In experiments undertaken in a pure science laboratory comparisons between methods are relatively easy. In biological experiments validity is less easy to assess and when the behavioural element becomes important it is particularly difficult to assess.

Reliability of a method is determined by repeating the experiment and measuring the ability of the method to produce consistent results. Again the reliability becomes progressively more difficult to assess objectively as the field of study moves from laboratory research to behavioural research.

Validity and reliability have to be checked at two main junctures of the research sequence. The first is the point at which information is collected and recorded and the second is the point at which it is classified and coded.

Some research methods and classifications have been widely used in the past and their validity and reliability confirmed by successful use. Many of the tests of personality and mood fall into this category and the advantages of using established methods when they are available and suitable are obvious. But the problems of research in general practice are increasingly calling for new methods of study (for example, direct observation by a third party, tape-recording or video-recording of consultation, simulation) and assessment of the quality of information collected using these techniques has to be individual to the project concerned. There are no ways of checking validity and reliability other than by repeating observations with the same and with different subjects and observers, and comparing results with those found using other methods. The research worker himself is best placed to know the strengths and weaknesses of the methods he is using and has a responsibility to reveal and measure the errors his methods may be causing.

Most of the errors introduced by different designs of research and methods of classification have already been referred to, and the only further point I wish to stress here is the need to remember the loss of reliability and validity caused by missing information. This is particularly important when considering retrospective research (analysis of practice records, for example) and when using replies to questionnaires where the response rate falls short of the total possible. It is unsafe to assume that non-responders and responders to questionnaires are the same kind of people or have had the same experiences and the greater the proportion of non-responders the less the confidence which can be placed in the representativeness and value of the information that is available. A carefully prepared postal questionnaire which includes a prepaid method for replying should attract a response from about two-thirds of those who receive it, and a reminder to non-responders should bring replies from a half to two-thirds of the remainder. By comparing the replies from the first and second questionnaires it is sometimes possible to evaluate the possible meaning of the remaining missing material.

In summary, checks have to be considered at the points of collecting information and classifying information. The first is often difficult; the second should be simpler. The decision on how much checking can and needs to be done is a matter for individual judgement. What is not in doubt is that any research report should discuss fully and frankly this important aspect of the interpretation of whatever results are being reported.

Statistical Significance

Suppose a bag containing a hundred sweets includes equal numbers coloured red, orange, green and yellow. If all aspects of the design of the sweets are identical there is a one in four chance that any sweet chosen will belong to say the red group, and a one in sixteen chance that two successive reds will be chosen, and a one in sixty-four chance that three successive reds will be chosen (provided of course that any sweet drawn is returned to the bag before the next sweet is drawn). The chances of any selected sequence or combination being drawn can be predicted and if sufficient attempts are made the predicted outcome will be met.

If, however, out of ten samples of three sweets taken from the full bag three orange sweets are found to be drawn together four times, what comment can be made on whether this represents a chance finding or alternatively means that the orange sweets belong to a different type of sweets than do the other colours (they might, for example, be heavier or stickier)?

Statistical tests are mathematical formulae which can be applied to numerical findings to allow comments to be made, for example, on:

(i) whether differences between observed and expected findings are likely to have arisen by chance;
(ii) whether associations that have been noted are likely to represent real relationships or coincidences;
(iii) whether the average values or distributions of findings in different samples suggest that the samples belong to the same population or represent parts of more than one population.

Statistical significance is a comment on the degree of probability that observed associations of whatever kind may have arisen through chance. By convention a probability (P) of findings occurring by chance not more than one time in twenty ($P \leqslant 0.05$ or 'significant at the five per cent level') is normally accepted as statistically significant; a probability of findings occurring not more than one time in a hundred ('significant at the one per cent level' or $P \leqslant 0.01$) is regarded as indicating that findings are 'statistically highly significant'.

The choice of which statistical test should, or should not, be applied depends on many factors including the number of observations made, the distribution of observations around their average value and whether, for example, numerical or verbal information forms the original basis for the numbers being analysed.

The pitfalls of the application of statistical tests are many. Gore *et al.* (BMJ, 1977) found an alarming number of errors both in the choice of statistical tests and the application of these tests in papers published in the *British Medical Journal.* Whenever possible professional statistical advice should be taken in preference to possibly ill-informed and thus misleading amateur help. For the reader wanting a more detailed introduction to the application of statistics to medical research Swinscow's *Statistics at Square One* and Bradford Hill's *Principles of Medical Statistics* are useful texts.

It is not my aim to provide a short cut to statistical competence; my intention is to explain some of the simple concepts relating to averages and distributions and comment briefly on two of the commoner statistical tests, the t-test and X^2 test (chi-squared).

Averages and Distributions

When a number of observations of a variable item are made (for example, 'duration of cough' in a group of patients treated with say DRUG A) these can be plotted on a graph or presented in a histogram as shown in Figure 12.1: the arithmetic 'mean' is the common 'average' obtained when the total value of all the observations is divided by the number of observations; the 'mode' is the number which occurs most frequently and the 'median' is the number which is found at the mid-point of the total number of observations. When observations are distributed in a completely balanced way around their mid-point as in Figure 12.1, the distribution is described as *normal*, and the mean, the median and the mode are the same.

If the distribution of days of duration of cough in a second group of 100 patients treated with DRUG B is asymmetrical as is shown in Figure 12.2, the distribution would be described as *skew* and the mean (5.2 days), median (5 days) and mode (4 days) would all differ.

Alternatively, observations may be distributed amongst categories as shown in Table 12.1. When information is presented in this way no comment can be made about the distributions of the observations, other than their relation to the point of division chosen for the table. The type of table shown in Table 12.1 is known as a 'fourfold' or

Figure 12.1: Duration of Cough (in days) in 68 Patients Treated with DRUG A

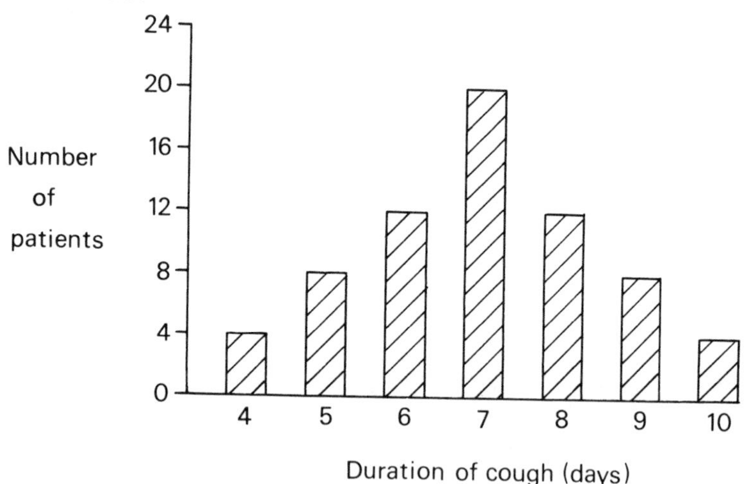

Figure 12.2: Duration of Cough (in days) in 100 Patients Treated with DRUG B

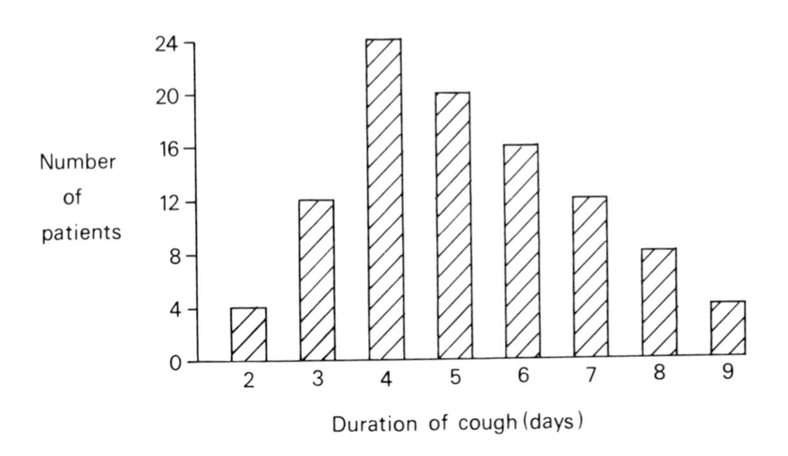

Table 12.1: Numbers of Patients Treated with DRUG A and DRUG B in Whom Cough Lasted Less Than 7 Days, or for 7 or More Days

	Duration of Cough	
	Less than 7 days	7 days or more
Patients receiving DRUG A	24	44
Patients receiving DRUG B	76	24

'2 x 2' table and is one of the commonest ways in which research findings are presented.

As an example of the restricted way in which it is possible to apply statistical tests, both the t-test and the X^2 test can be applied to the distributions shown in Figures 12.1 and 12.2 which have symmetrical distributions and are unimodal (that is, have a single peak). The X^2 test but *not* the t-test can be applied to information distributed in any other way, or in an unknown way, as is the case in the analysis shown in

Table 12.1.

The t-test

If in Figure 12.3 the line C-C is the distribution of days of cough in a sample of 50 patients treated with DRUG C and line D-D is the same distribution for 50 patients treated with DRUG D, the t-test is designed to allow comment to be made on whether patients treated with DRUG C and DRUG D represent samples from the same or different populations.

If these two groups of 50 patients were initially drawn as two samples from the same population, and now appear to belong to different populations, then either the samples were not random, or some new factor has been introduced which makes them different – such as the difference between DRUG C and DRUG D.

The t-test is basically a comparison of the *means* of the samples being studied. However, two samples may have the same mean but widely different (although both symmetrical) distributions as shown in Figure 12.4, and the t-test can only be applied if the shape of the distribution in the two samples is similar. The shape of the distribution

Figure 12.3: Distribution of Days Duration of Cough in 50 Patients Treated with DRUG C (line C-C) and 50 Patients Treated with DRUG D (line D-D)

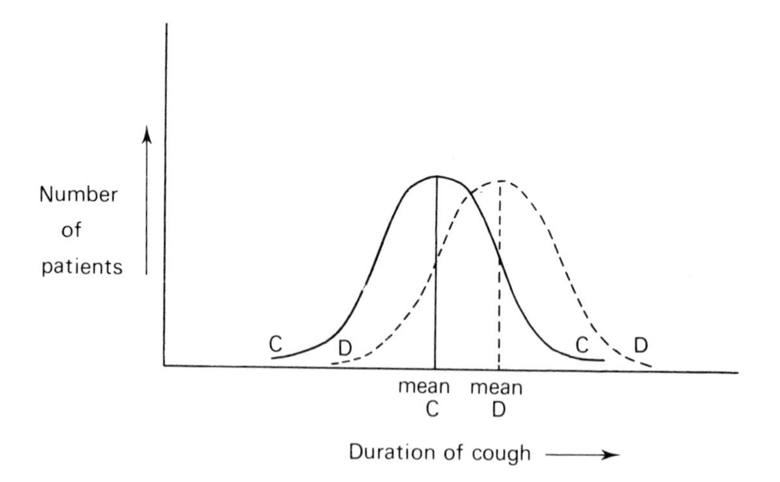

Figure 12.4: Different Possible Distributions of Samples with the Same Mean

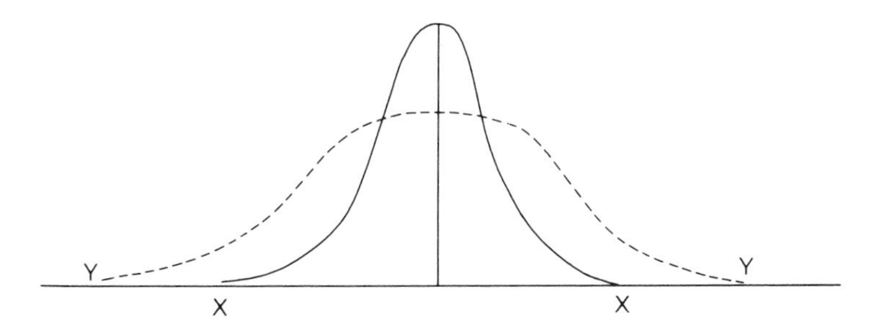

X-X or Y-Y is known as the *variance* which is a specially calculated statistic, the square root of which is known as the *standard deviation.* The t-test requires that the means being compared are from samples with similar variances.

In a normal distribution, approximately two-thirds of observations will lie within plus or minus one standard deviation of the mean of the sample, approximately 95 per cent of observations will lie within two standard deviations, and approximately 99 per cent within three standard deviations.

The X^2 Test

The X^2 test can be applied to many different kinds of observations but the example of the 2 x 2 table shown in Table 12.1 is the easiest to develop. The test depends on measuring the difference between the expected and the observed frequency distributions in each 'cell' of the table. The influence of the size of the sample studied in producing differences of real significance between observed and expected numbers is allowed for in the mathematical formula used. For any box or cell in a table, $X^2 = \frac{(O\text{-}E)^2}{E}$ where E is the expected number and O the observed number. If the example introduced in Table 12.1 is re-examined, the four cells can each be given an identifying letter a, b, c or d, as follows:

	24 a	b 44
	c 76	d 24

68 patients received DRUG A and 100 DRUG B; 100 patients have no cough by the seventh day, and 68 are still coughing at the seventh day. If there is no difference between the effectiveness of treatment A and treatment B, the 168 patients should be distributed as follows:

	Duration of Cough				
	Less than 7 days		7 days or more		Total
Patients receiving DRUG A	40.5	a	b	27.5	68
Patients receiving DRUG B	59.5	c	d	40.5	100
Total	100			68	168

From this stage the value for X^2 for each cell and thus for the whole table can be calculated using the formula shown above. When X^2 is calculated for a 2 x 2 table, if X^2 is 3.84 or greater the difference between observed and expected frequences is significant at the 5 per cent level ($P \leqslant 0.05$), that is, unlikely to have arisen by chance more often than once in twenty tests, samples or observations (a X^2 of 6.63 or more indicates significance at the 1 per cent or one in a hundred level). Special variations of the X^2 test require to be used when either the total numbers are small or when any one box or cell contains a small expected or observed number; any figure of below 20 in one cell will usually require application of modifications to the standard X^2 test.

X^2 estimations must always be carried out on absolute numbers; never on percentages.

The Null Hypothesis

The term null hypothesis is given to a hypothesis which proposes that there will be

> no real differences between samples being compared and that they may be assumed to have been drawn from *one* population; or
> that there will be no real difference between observed and expected findings; or
> that there will be no real correlation between sets of observations.

The null hypothesis cannot be proved true; it can only be rejected as unlikely to be true if significant differences between the samples, or expected and observed distributions, are found. Thus, when the null hypothesis is rejected the conclusion is that it is likely that there are significant differences between samples, or between observed and expected findings, and an alternative hypothesis can then be advanced to account for these findings and, if appropriate, tested separately.

Statistical tests properly applied to reliable and valid material will enhance the insight with which results are interpreted. Wrongly applied to poor material they do nothing but harm the reputation of the user; they certainly do not improve what has gone before!

Clinical Significance

Even after good-quality information has been submitted to the correct tests of statistical significance, there remain two possible weaknesses in the fact that *statistical significance* only mirrors probability or chance. One is incorrectly attributing significance which is not real, the other is failing to recognise real differences which are present despite apparent lack of statistical significance. The first weakness is especially likely to arise when multiple analyses are undertaken; because significance at the usual level of 5 per cent implies that there is one chance in twenty of the finding occurring by chance, when twenty comparisons are made it is likely that one 'significant' finding will arise simply because of the definition of significance. Two hundred comparisons will produce ten 'significant' findings and so on. But these significances are technical and not a safe basis for stating *clinical* conclusions. In short, statistical significance does not automatically imply clinical significance. When 'statistical significance' is observed during multiple testing as part of a 'to see what we can find' approach, it is probably safer to use this as the starting point for testing a hypothesis based on the identified association.

The opposite possibility is that a clinically important difference between two sets of observations may fail to reach the conventional level of statistical significance either by chance or because the size of the study has been too small. Adding together several small studies (the basis of the multi-centre study) may create significance which would be missed otherwise; the risk of course is that unlike observations or unlike samples are incorrectly aggregated. And, again, at the end of the process we have to ask if a finding that requires enormous samples to produce statistical significance is in reality capable of being clinically significant.

Those interested in reading more about the difficulties of balancing clinical and statistical significance will find the *British Medical Journal* (1977) correspondence involving Dudley, Peto & Doll and St John-Brooks of value. Peto & Doll put the case against 'over-slavish adherence to rigid criteria of statistical significance' and St John-Brooks draws attention to the attendant introduction of a 'far from negligible element of subjective judgement into interpretation of observed results'. He suggests that probability statistics are 'of use for guidance, support and restraint'. It is the balancing of the concepts of statistical and clinical significance that provides the art of research interpretation, in particular in the more behavioural areas of research that general practice research inevitably involves.

Beware of. . .

Before leaving this section on interpretation of findings, I want to draw attention to a number of techniques which are sometimes used in presenting results and which may mislead an observer attempting to assess research reports. Some, such as converting 'days' to 'hours' to produce larger and superficially more impressive numbers, are relatively harmless and merely serve to emphasise how necessary it is that the assessment of clinical significance should be seen as a separate stage in interpreting research.

Others, frequently on display at medical meetings, in journals and during visits from pharmaceutical representatives, are more subtle. The capacity to distort information is an educational skill in itself and I want here only to hint at some of the possibilities that the critic or reader should look out for.

Reference Lists

It is common to quote as references 'personal communications', 'unpublished work', quotations from 'papers presented at International symposia' and material 'on file', giving the impression that findings are well documented. This is unfair practice as it creates a false impression of the intellectual solidarity of the material being presented. When offered a reference list be duly suspicious of this kind of approach, particularly if the references are concentrated in unknown journals, are all written by one author especially if of uncertain standing, or are published in foreign languages.

Truncated Histograms

Use of a histogram bearing only the upper portion of a scale is perhaps the easiest way of creating a false visual image. In the left half of Figure 12.5 there would appear to be little difference between the effectiveness of hypnotics A and B; when the histogram is truncated as shown in the right half of the figure, the false impression is created

Figure 12.5: Distortion of Visual Impact Caused by Truncating a Histogram

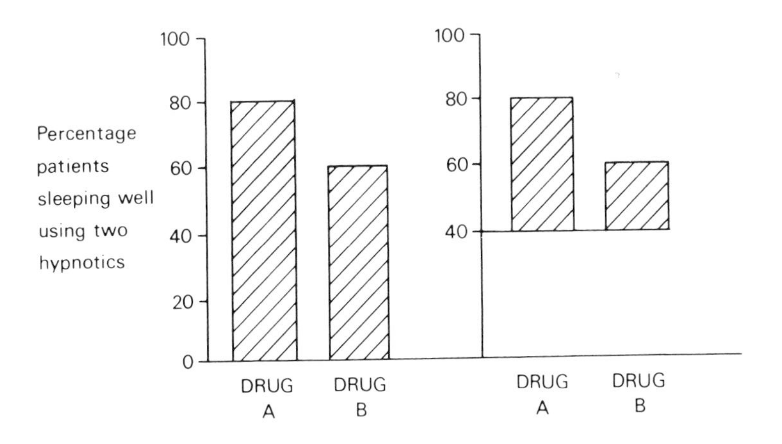

that DRUG A is twice as effective as DRUG B.

Selected Scales

Changing the scale of an X- or Y- axis in a graph or histogram can also greatly alter the visual impact. Figure 12.6 shows the length of time to recovery of patients on a particular treatment.

The visual impact is again substantially changed and greater alteration would have been achieved by, for example, doubling the scale on the Y-axis at the same time. The use of logarithmic scales can be particularly effective in this way.

Beware of speakers who gloss over the scales in their graphs and the absolute numbers behind their percentages when presenting visual material.

Absent controls

It is common to be presented with results of observations 'before' and 'after' treatment with a particular drug, and be given no accompanying graphs or information on control patients observed for the same period of time but not on treatment. This is particularly common in reports on the effectiveness of antibiotics, psychotropic drugs and hypotensive

Figure 12.6: Weeks to Recovery Plotted Against Patients Studied

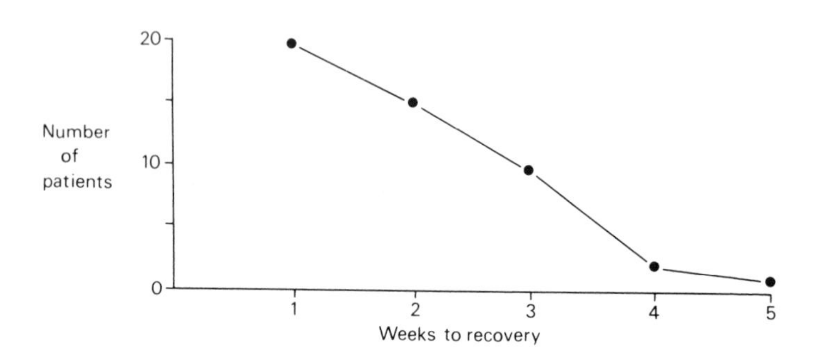

Figure 12.7: Some Information as in Figure 12.6; Scale on X-axis Halved

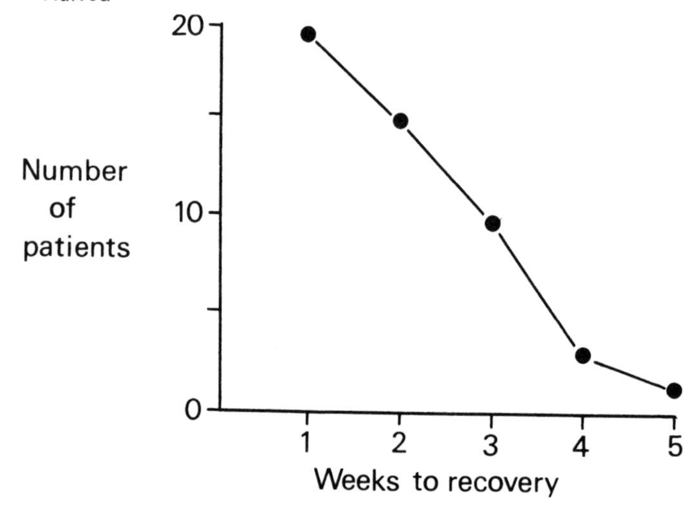

agents, and often the trends illustrated could be representing no more than the natural history of the untreated illness. Figure 12.8 demonstrates the visual effectiveness of this kind of incomplete information.

Figure 12.8: Average Blood Pressure in a Group of Patients Before and After Two Weeks' Treatment on DRUG A

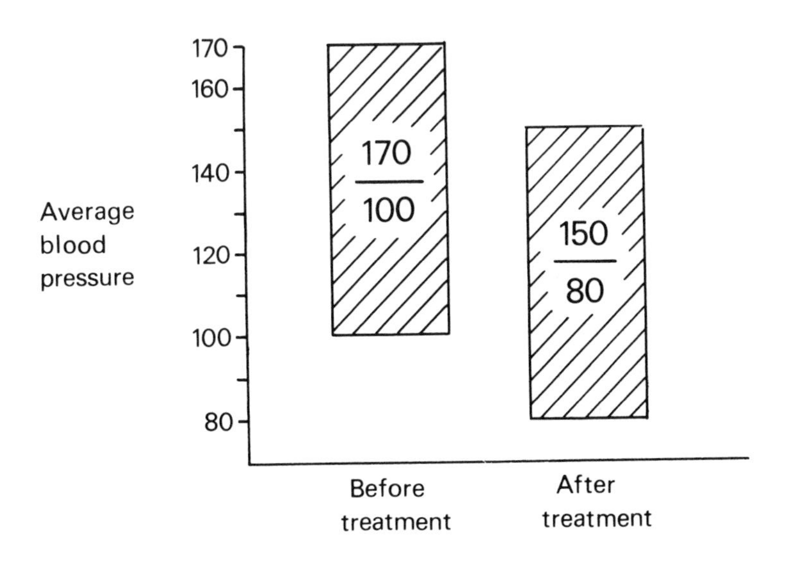

Misquotation

Regrettably scientific work is from time to time quoted out of context and thereby presented in a quite misleading manner. This misdemeanour may even include constructing inappropriate visual displays out of numerical statistics and adding in small print '. . .adapted from. . .' the work of accepted authorities.

Scientific Overkill

Highly complex graphs and tables littered with Greek symbols, arrows, figures and so on may represent an attempt to pre-empt technical and scientific debate. Ask for simplification – it is not always forthcoming!

Any thoughtful reader knows the favourable impression created by an entertaining speaker, a well-written paper or skilled advertising. Always be sure that the scientific components of a message are assessed as science separately, and maintain a courteous but probing scepticism – learn to ask questions routinely and regularly:

how was the information collected?
how was the quality of the information checked?
what statistical tests were used?
have they been correctly interpreted?
what is the clinical significance of the findings and conclusions presented?

References

Dudley, H.A.F., 'When is Significant not Significant?', *British Medical Journal*, 2 (1977), p.47.

Gore, S.M., Jones, I.G. & Rytter, E.C., 'Misuse of Statistical Methods: Critical Assessment of Articles in BMJ from January to March 1976', *British Medical Journal*, 1 (1977), pp.85-7.

Hill, A.B., *Principles of Medical Statistics*, 9th edn. (The Lancet, London, 1971).

Peto, R. & Doll, R., 'When is Significant not Significant?', *British Medical Journal*, 2 (1977), p.259.

St John-Brooks, W.H., 'When is Significant not Significant?', *British Medical Journal*, 2 (1977), p.386.

Swinscow, T.D.V., *Statistics at Square One* (British Medical Journal, London, 1976).

13 SUCCESSES AND DISAPPOINTMENTS

This chapter concludes a sequence which has taken us from asking questions, through the development of ideas and the design and organisation of projects, to the analysis and interpretation of results. The six projects introduced as examples of research in Chapters 6 and 10 were left unfinished at the stage of analysing and commenting on the findings, and I want in this chapter to present briefly the conclusions of these studies and to make some comments on the strengths and weaknesses of the projects.

Project One: 'Early or Late Antibiotics in a Flu Epidemic?' (continued from page 108)

Four hundred and forty-eight courses of tetracycline and 388 courses of placebo were taken. The principal results of the study are summarised in Table 13.1.

The average duration of purulent sputum recorded for the illnesses treated with the antibiotic was 2.3 days; in 60 per cent of the illnesses no purulent sputum developed and in 6 per cent purulent sputum persisted ten days or more. Work loss averaged 1.1 days per illness, and 3 per cent of the illnesses required treatment with a different antibiotic. 6.7 per cent of patients developed side-effects during treatment.

Table 13.1: Comparison of Outcome Between Tetracycline and Placebo Takers

	Tetracycline takers	Placebo takers
Number of patients	448	388
Average days' purulent sputum recorded per illness	2.3	2.6
% illness in which purulent sputum developed	60	59
% illness in which purulent sputum lasted 10 days or more	6	7
Days' work loss per illness	1.1	1.5
% patients developing side effects	6.7	1.8
% patients requiring treatment with different antibiotic	3	5

For the patients who took the placebo the average duration of purulent sputum recorded was 2.6 days; 59 per cent illnesses remained free of purulent sputum and in 7 per cent its presence persisted ten days or more. Work loss averaged 1.5 days per illness, 5 per cent of illnesses required an antibiotic and 1.8 per cent of patients reported side-effects.

In short, there was no evidence of benefit in being an antibiotic taker; the almost four-fold increase in side-effects, although falling short of statistical significance, provided some evidence that patients had complied with instructions on medication. (Compliance with medication is difficult to assess without measuring blood levels and this is, of course, rarely feasible in general practice research. Drugs which, for example, alter the colour of the urine are a rare assistance to solving this problem. Pill counts are helpful when the pills are present, but the absence of pills does not necessarily mean that they have been taken as directed.)

Numerous sub-divisions of the results were possible. Patients were divided into three age-groups by decade; there were non-smokers, light and heavy smokers; individual symptoms were studied in relation to whether they developed before or after treatment was started. Results for each of the six months of the study were examined separately. For each sub-group of patients the outcome on active treatment was compared with the outcome on placebo treatment and out of over 50 chi-squared tests, none suggested advantage to antibiotic takers.

The large number of illnesses studied, the fact that 92 per cent of record cards were returned, the random sampling to antibiotic and placebo groups and double-blind design all provided reassurance that biases resulting from the design of the trial were likely to have been kept to a minimum. In some of the sub-divisions of the results the smallness of numbers available made us reluctant to accept the negative conclusions as necessarily real. Of particular interest was the finding that 44 patients who started tetracycline after development of purulent sputum fared no better than 35 who started placebo at the same stage of illness. Although this suggested that patients with the symptom of purulent sputum may not benefit from antibiotic treatment it seemed wiser to use this finding as a justification for a further and larger study rather than as an unsupported basis for determining clinical policy (Stott & West (1976) have since confirmed the lack of benefit of antibiotic use in treatment of normally healthy patients presenting with purulent sputum).

Also of interest was the high incidence of prolonged purulent sputum in both antibiotic and placebo takers in November and December (8 per cent and 11 per cent of patients respectively) as compared with March and April (4 per cent and 3 per cent of patients respectively). Had the treatments been compared consecutively instead of simultaneously it would have appeared that either antibiotic or placebo worked better depending on which had been tried second. How often we hear of personal prescribing policies being determined on this very kind of 'evidence'!

If we accept that patients did take their tablets as they were asked to and as they indicated they had done, and that they recorded their clinical progress accurately (any recording errors which did take place should have been equally distributed between antibiotic and placebo takers), the conclusions from the study must lie between the following extremes:

> antibiotics do not help treatment of minor respiratory illness; and
> this particular antibiotic, prescribed in this way during the winter concerned in the part of Glasgow studied, did not help normally healthy male patients aged 20 to 49 in terms of. . .

In retrospect my assessment of the contribution made by this study is simply that it provides some evidence which helps the development of an antibiotic prescribing policy for general practice respiratory illness. It did not prove anything because it was not designed to. Even if nothing else, 388 patients who received placebo came to no harm and only 5 per cent of them received an antibiotic later in their illness. Of course, it is impossible to say how many of these patients would have come to the doctor had the trial not been taking place, but none the less this kind of evidence supports the view that a conservative approach to managing minor respiratory illness is tenable. Since being involved in this study, I have prescribed fewer antibiotics early in the course of flu-like illnesses and no longer routinely prescribe antibiotics to normally healthy patients simply because they have purulent sputum.

Project Two: 'Do "Diagnoses" Determine or Justify Management Decisions?' (continued from page 112)

Sixty-two doctors used 119 diagnostic labels to describe 7,515 new episodes of illness; they prescribed antibiotics to 68 per cent of patients. Some diagnostic labels (for example, tracheitis) were frequently used in some group practices, but never in others. Other terms (for example, pharyngitis and tonsillitis) appeared to be used almost interchangeably. Apparently similar illnesses were labelled with terms which have significantly different implications – the 16 terms used to describe illnesses characterised by crepitations or rhonchi in the chest were labelled as anything from pneumonia and bronchitis, to coryza, URTI and influenza.

In short, 73 per cent of patients had illnesses which belonged to a symptom/sign complex able to predict four times out of five whether antibiotics would be prescribed; but only 55 per cent of patients had a diagnostic label attached which was equally able to predict whether antibiotic treatment would be used. My hypothesis that in the context of new episodes of respiratory illness 'there would be a better correlation between *clinical information collected* and *treatment given* than between *clinical information collected* and *diagnosis made* or between *diagnosis made* and *treatment given*' was clearly supported. It could be argued that the doctors who took part had been biased by the briefing they received, or were unrepresentative of doctors generally. I can only claim to have carefully avoided introducing bias during my early discussions with the doctors and none who took part have suggested they were primed – in any case the pretence would have been difficult to sustain during six months of a busy winter. The 62 doctors chosen were unrepresentative in that most had teaching commitments, but they formed 25 per cent of the doctors in the administrative area of the local Health Board, represented all but three of those approached and more recruits could without doubt have been found if necessary. I was content to identify those doctors as representative of the kind of doctor with whom I would be happy to see my family registered – a reasonable way of closing debate on this issue!

What of the possibility that the information collected using my questionnaire was not reliable or not valid? It is always difficult to defend new methods of study and in the end a reasonable assessment of available subjective and objective evidence may be all that is possible. Forty-two of the 62 doctors had taken part in a different study involving listing diagnostic labels and drugs prescribed two years previously. A high consistency of diagnostic labelling and antibiotic prescribing was noted for these doctors between the two studies. A direct-observer study of local doctors at work and an interview study of diagnostic and prescribing habits in respiratory illness (both involving a proportion of the doctors who took part in this current study) suggested consistency between all three studies in relation to percentages of patients in whom throat, chest and ears were apparently examined, temperatures taken or no examination carried out. The average number of symptoms and signs indicated in this current study as determining clinical policy (seven) was the same as that found in the interview study mentioned above. And students attached to the practices during recording periods confirmed that the forms had been completed as conscientiously as appeared to be the case. I also felt that the willingness of doctors to return consistently high numbers of forms throughout a six-month study and to reflect the peak of influenzal illness with a peak of research returns was the highest possible indication of good faith on their part.

If the method seems defensible, and the hypothesis is seen to be numerically supportable, what of its clinical importance? I had hoped to be able to say that my evidence proved that, in given circumstances, doctors make management decisions first and then add diagnostic labels to justify their management decisions. Although I still believe this to be true and my evidence is compatible with such a conclusion, I have to realise that as much as I can claim to have shown in this study is:

> that when management and diagnostic decisions are entered on a record it cannot be assumed that the two are related in the sequence diagnosis —> management.

But even this has profound implications for all retrospective record-based research: and much of general practice research belongs to this category.

There was, of course, much more to be taken from analysis of this study, and it was important to decide at what point the accuracy of the information fell below the quality necessary for conclusions to be drawn. It is sad how often the impact of a valuable study is lost because the investigator does not sense when to stop squeezing his information. Most well-conceived studies will produce enough possible associations of findings to start off several new investigations and that is the best way to use information of uncertain credibility.

Project Three: 'Co-trimoxazole and Streptococcal Tonsillitis'
(continued from page 115)

As a clinical trial comparing the merits of co-trimoxazole and penicillin in streptococcal tonsillitis this project had already sunk without trace! Ultimately this was because doctors were selecting patients for the different treatments and not allocating to each test group in a properly random manner. My responsibility for this error had been in not insisting on a double-blind design. I also now realise that the aims of the study had not included a statement of what would have been taken as a clinically significant difference between the two groups of patients.

But it is a rare study from which nothing can be salvaged! Thirteen patients with beta-haemolytic streptococcal isolates received a week's penicillin and were swabbed at the end of four weeks. Five cultures were again positive. If the original paper suggesting why ten days' penicillin is preferable to five days' is consulted (Wannamaker *et al.*, 1953) it will be seen that this poor clearance rate almost exactly repeats the earlier figure for the five days' penicillin course. Seven days' would not appear to be a bacteriologically acceptable compromise between the five-day course and the ten-day course (which we suspect is rarely taken as directed).

The second bonus was the opportunity to study the use of patient reply cards as a method of assessing adverse reactions to drugs. The patients on penicillin provided a control for the method used and patients on (high-dose) co-trimoxazole represented the test group. Leaving aside gastro-intestinal and non-specific side-effects, no rashes were found in 55 penicillin takers as against eight rashes in 58 co-trimoxazole takers. A short paper was prepared drawing attention to this finding and pointing out that this method of patient follow-up had allowed the identification of side-effects which would otherwise have either not been reported by the patients or not recognised by the doctors. The paper was not accepted for publication for a variety of reasons, ranging from the essentially negative clinical findings also reported in it, to understandable but arguable concern that to use high doses of co-trimoxazole for this clinical indication had been wrong. (Earlier work in this region had shown that several general practitioners routinely used co-trimoxazole for what they diagnosed as tonsillitis, and we believed that this provided a reasonable defence against this criticism.) However, one reason quoted was that one referee did not believe the incidence of side-effects reported, giving the opinion that 'gastro-intestinal side-effects. . .are not usually complained of from this drug', and concluding that the study and methods used were 'quite unfair to' co-trimoxazole! Even 'evidence' is, it seems, a relative concept.

(The relevant information was eventually published in the correspondence columns of the *British Medical Journal* under the heading 'Drug Monitoring and Adverse Reactions' (1977).)

Project Four: 'The Prevention of Adverse Drug Reactions' (continued from page 117)

1,218 drugs were prescribed at least once to the 153 patients whose records had been tagged with the anticoagulant interaction warning labels which were under test in this study. No new prescriptions for barbiturates and only five new prescriptions for other drugs listed on the warning label had been issued.

1,264 drugs had been prescribed at least once to the 148 patients whose records had not been tagged and were acting as controls. Four new barbiturate prescriptions had been issued (by four different doctors in the group of 68 responsible for these patients) and twelve new prescriptions for other drugs on the test warning label.

The difference in potentially interacting prescriptions of five against sixteen was found to be statistically significant at the five per cent level. The report of the study accepted that recording of information was likely 'not to be entirely accurate' but assumed that errors should have applied equally to test and control groups. The clinical implications drawn were modest: '. . .that the simple system described goes some way to contribute to the reduction in the unintentional initiation of preventable adverse drug interactions in patients on outpatient anticoagulant therapy'. The results of the study, although encouraging, were barely sufficient to allow us to claim that the system was of real clinical value.

Fifteen patients had died during the six months between start and finish of the recording period. 'Value' for the system would perhaps have been proved had the deaths been attributable to interactions and found significantly more often in the control group. (The only death possibly attributable to interaction did occur in a patient in the control group.)

The question asked was simple, the project design simple; analysis was done by hand and interpretation was simple. Because of the limited clinical material available within the region in which we had the necessary access to records, only limited objectives were realistic. This is often the case when research is undertaken within a practice or group of practices. It is better to recognise and work within such limitations than to aim for unrealistic goals; this second course is an unerring recipe for failure and frustration and is one of the commonest reasons for disillusionment among inexperienced researchers.

Project Five: 'Can Clinical Judgement Be Analysed?' (continued from page 124)

Of the 1,000 booklets containing photographs of inflamed throats which were posted to general practitioners, 634 were returned within one month and analysed. Forty-one replies were blank, being from doctors who had retired, were not in general practice or had misgivings about the design of the study or the quality of the reproductions.

The 593 usable replies were in the form of YES or NO responses to twelve questions, 'Would you prescribe an antibiotic to patient 1-12?' For each 'patient', half the respondents were replying to one question, while the remaining respondents had been asked a slightly different question, but shown the same picture. A code on the reply card indicated which combination of questions had been included in each booklet.

The results were easily analysed by hand and twelve tables of which the one below is typical were constructed:

	Antibiotic 'prescribed'		
	YES	NO	
Patient details			
University student	69 (23%)	231	300
University student due to sit exams next week	202 (69%)	91	293
	271	322	593

$x^2 > 6.63$ $P < 0.01$

In six of the twelve tables differences significant at the $P < 0.01$ level were found, and in a seventh a difference significant at the $P < 0.05$ level was found. In five tables non-significant differences were found.

The hypothesis 'that awareness of non-physical features in a consultation may influence in a measurable way the doctor's decision to prescribe a physical remedy' had certainly been demonstrated to be true in the setting used for the study. Two main criticisms of the method had to be answered before discussing the relevance of the findings. First, it was necessary to consider whether the answers on the reply cards reflected clinical practice. This issue is the same as was discussed earlier in this chapter for project two and the best defence of the method is that the responses accurately mirrored the known diversity of prescribing habits of doctors seeing patients with inflamed throats. The method, of course, should also have been equally fallible for the test and control groups which had been designed to differ in psychological history only.

This leads to the second possible criticism, that colour intensity might have changed during printing, leading to one group of reproductions attracting different responses as a result. The four 'colour control' patients (numbers 1, 6, 12 and 15, in the booklet – see page 120) had been included to measure this risk. The 593 replies belonged to six different sets of combinations of the test patient histories. Approximately 100 replies had been received for each set, and the replies relating to the 'colour control' patients showed a consistent rate of YES and NO replies for each of the six sets. It therefore seemed reasonable to exclude variation in colour intensity as a source of bias.

A final support for the validity of the method was found when the original transparencies relating to the patients were projected to two audiences totalling 60 doctors, with the histories used in the study overprinted on the photographs and the order mixed. The same differences were found between the replies to the alternative histories for the same picture, the control patients continued to be answered consistently, and the YES percentages for test and control patients were remarkably similar to those obtained using the printed booklets.

My original aim had been to demonstrate numerically how 'patient' factors influence the clinical decisions taken by general practitioners; the motive behind this was my wish to demonstrate that the philosophy of general practice differs from that of hospital medicine in the relatively greater importance which general practitioners attach to patient against illness factors in taking clinical decisions in the context of illness seen outside hospital. Demonstration of this difference seems to me an important part of preparing the defence of the right of the general practitioner to determine his own clinical identity and to be left as the principal arbiter of acceptable quality of care within his own field of work. It is also, of course, an important aid to arguing why general practice should have an independent role in the teaching of medical students.

No hospital specialist who has seen my material has suggested he would prescribe antibiotics to more than a small minority of my 'patients'. I suppose this is technically not enough evidence to allow me to consider my case proven. But on this occasion I feel that the onus is on anyone who feels that I have not proved my case to produce his facts in support of the alternative hypothesis.

Project Six: 'Prescribing to Save Work' (continued from page 126)

When the records of the 153 patients who had been selected for the study were examined for the period 1970-6 a total of 856 apparently discrete episodes of respiratory illness were identified. Each was allocated to the doctor who had carried out the first consultation, whose (apparent) antibiotic prescribing policy for new respiratory illness was then calculated. The frequency with which a change of antibiotic or the introduction of an antibiotic was required within two weeks of the first consultation was noted and attributed as a 'failure' to the doctor who had made the first consultation. Over all, all the five doctors (aggregating successive trainees into a hypothetical single trainee) had similar failure rates (average 6 per cent, range 5-8 per cent) although their rate of use of antibiotics for first consultations ranged from 48 per cent to 88 per cent.

The number of new consultations for respiratory illness which would have been expected if the figures in the National Morbidity Study of 1974 were accepted as a norm would have been 650 as against the 856 found. The apparent excess over expectation was 31 per cent.

These simple findings are objective to the degree with which it can be accepted that what has been recorded did take place and was all that took place. Further sub-divisions based on clinical details would have been impossible to validate partly because of the difficulty of assessing whether absent information was negative or not elicited, and partly because standard interpretations of positive information would have been unlikely. Consultation with the doctor, field of illness, and prescription or not of an antibiotic on the other hand are relatively likely to be accurately reported, particularly as the practice policy was to take records on house calls and to record details of out-of-hours calls. Inevitably records of some consultations will not have been entered; a judgement has to be made of how many, what kind and how crucial to the study. Our view was that the missing information would have been unlikely to influence the findings to a significant degree, but our conclusions are again stated cautiously because of the unavoidable uncertainty over the quality of data available. We concluded only that there was 'absence of any support for the belief that prescribing antibiotics on a large scale saves work' and noted that 'an above average practice antibiotic prescribing frequency appears associated with an above average respiratory illness consultation rate'.

Other analyses in which the children and adults were considered separately and the 'failed' cases were examined in greater detail to attempt to recognise doctor, patient or illness influences were of interest but nothing conclusive was found. The patients who had consulted most had received most antibiotics and were readily recognised as including many belonging to the 'problem families' of the practice. Is there a correlation between prescribing rates of antibiotics to children and psychotropics to their mothers. . .? And so the research sequence starts again.

Four of these six projects were analysed by hand, one using a counter-sorter and one with the aid of the computer. No statistical tests were used in project three, only X^2 tests in projects one, four, five and six, and only X^2 tests and a test of correlation in project two. A great deal of evidence was collected and much of it used only to prepare the background for further studies, to support teaching and indirectly to influence attitudes to patient care. Simple questions were asked and most were answered, at least in part. Where hypotheses were tested, interpretation of results was easier. Conclusions claimed for the research were relatively few; the implications of the research were hopefully more far-reaching.

Nothing described in the three chapters which have outlined these projects throughout their development was in any way difficult to understand – not even mathematically. Given a question of interest, time to consider its implications and a logical and practical plan to investigate an aspect of the issue, research is an activity well within the scope of all general practitioners; it is also an activity which, even if it may be time-consuming, can add interest to a job which may have become routine and sharpness to a mind which may have become uncritical. It can even make Monday morning a time for expectation instead of foreboding!

References

Howie, J.G.R., 'Drug Monitoring and Adverse Reactions', *British Medical Journal*, 1 (1977), p.1467.

Stott, N.C.H. & West, R.R., 'Randomised Controlled Trial of Antibiotics in Patients with Cough and Purulent Sputum', *British Medical Journal*, 2 (1976), pp.556-9.

Wannamaker, L.W. *et al.*, 'The Effect of Penicillin Prophylaxis on Streptococcal Disease Rates and the Carrier State', *New England Journal of Medicine*, 249 (1953), pp.1-7.

PART FOUR

TELLING ABOUT RESEARCH

14 WRITING ABOUT RESEARCH

No matter how successful or unsuccessful a project may seem to have been it is always helpful to commit a summary of it to paper for discussion. It is helpful (as well as being a matter of common courtesy) to show such a document, or sometimes a modified form of it, to those who have either helped in the design of the project or made information available. In addition, if funding has been provided the body concerned will expect to see a report of how it has been used. The research worker himself can focus on whether his initial aims have been met, and writing a report helps sharpen the conclusions which are drawn from the work. Errors can be identified, lessons learned, and future possibilities for research brought to the surface. Finally, those for whom a study may have implications (for example, one's partners) should be encouraged to look critically at the design, results and interpretation of the work before accepting or rejecting its conclusions.

By the time the processes of analysis and interpretation have begun most researchers will have a reasonable idea of how the final report on the project is to be laid out. A report will normally be between 1,500 and 2,000 words in length and comprise an introduction, sections on methods, results and discussion of the results, and end with (or alternatively be prefaced by) a summary.

The introduction (around 300 words) explains the background to the study and ends with a statement of the aims of the study. It will include relevant references to published work but should not be used as a demonstration of how widely one has read. This section describes the *why* and *what* of the project. The second section will describe the methods used for the study and should describe in some detail how doctors, patients, illnesses or whatever were selected for the study and any reasons for excluding participants from the study. Laboratory techniques or questionnaires should be described or references to established methods quoted. This section will be rather longer (perhaps 500 words) and describes the *how* of the project.

The results section, usually about the same length as the methods section, presents the findings of the study. Care should be taken to avoid introducing further description of method (other than techniques used to handle the data) and discussion of the significance of the results should be left to the next section. It is helpful to summarise the principal positive and negative findings in a small number (not more than three or four) of well-headed, clear tables. Subsidiary analyses, particularly when describing negative findings, can be covered by a general statement along the lines '. . .no differences were found when patients were divided into age groups, marital status. . .' It is not necessary to restate the details of the tables in the text, but correct to emphasise the key findings. Figures should be trimmed of irrelevant decimal points and the use of percentages watched with great care especially when dealing with numbers below about 30 or 40. Graphs or histograms may help demonstrate findings not easily summarised in text or tables; the scales on the axes must be clearly stated. Statistical tests used should be stated in sufficient detail to allow the reader to check their appropriateness.

If the results section represents *what was found*, the discussion section represents *what does it mean* and *what should happen next.* Comment should be made on the validity and reliability of the techniques used and on the clinical as well as the statistical significance of the findings. The final paragraph should outline future developments suggested by the study or apparently necessary to confirm possible, but not certain findings. This section should normally be no longer than that describing methods or results.

The final part, often attached as the front page of a research report, is the summary. The summary may be the only part of a report which will be read, and great care should be taken to ensure that it has the desired impact. It should be short but informative; it is a mistake to make it so brief that the main points of the study are obscured. At the end of the report appropriate acknowledgement should be made of help received and all references quoted in the text listed in an approved style.

So far, I have avoided equating the preparation of a research report (which should be encouraged as a routine) with publishing a research paper, which should depend on having something to say which has a relevance to a wider audience. Usually the message will be a positive one but sometimes a negative finding has greater importance than might be realised. Preparing a thesis for a higher degree is another activity in the field of writing which deserves thought. A thesis will bring together a series of projects which develop one theme to a greater depth than is usually possible in a single project. Writing a thesis should be seen as an exercise which develops powers of criticism, deduction and perseverance (all relevant to the work of teachers and practising physicians) rather than as simply the acquisition of a further registrable qualification!

Whatever is written should at least be readable and preferably interesting and understandable as well. The principal rules for good scientific writing are simple. Use well-constructed short sentences; use simple words when simple words are available; and use as few words as are necessary to convey the meaning you want. Much has been written on how to write and the reader looking for advice should browse through the classic *Thorne's Better Medical Writing.*

Writing for Publication

Most general practitioners who attempt to write scientific articles make mistakes which they could avoid by 'doing their homework' a little more thoroughly. Advice from more experienced writers is rarely hard to find and a few weeks spent getting a paper right makes a substantial difference to the chances of its being accepted by a hard-pressed journal editor.

First check that you have a message which is able to sustain an original article; if not, consider writing a 'short report' or making a contribution to the correspondence columns when a suitable leader or other paper gives an opening. Choose a journal which publishes papers which are similar in style to the one you are preparing and attempt to slant your introduction (and later covering letter) to recent issues raised in the journal's columns. Three or four apt and up-to-date references are usually to be preferred to a patchy out-of-date dip into the archives of medical folklore.

If instructions for authors are available, read and act on them. If, for example, 'short reports' have to be of no more than 600 words, do not offer 700! Look at the journal's policy on tables and graphs and the way references are normally presented.

When you have written your paper (modelled for general purposes on the 1,500-word report described above) leave it a week or two and read it again. You will probably be horrified at its lack of conciseness and clarity, the non-sequiturs it contains, its gaps in logic and its grammatical shortcomings. Correct these weaknesses and ask two or three colleagues to approve the new version. Consider their comments thoughtfully, make any final changes and send it to the journal you have chosen.

My own habit has been to include a short covering note explaining why I am asking the particular journal to consider the article for publication, but not all authors believe this is necessary or appropriate.

Some journals respond quickly, others less quickly, and some take a quite unjustifiably long time – so long in fact that I would think twice before letting them have a manuscript. Your advisers will help you to decide where to try first. No writer of any experience has all his papers accepted and sometimes those that are rejected seem better than others which appear in print. Having a paper turned down is always disappointing; it may be that the rejection is a consequence of the shortage of journal space, or of the current priorities of a particular journal or of editorial preferences and frailties. Quite frequently reasons for rejection are given; although the first reaction is often to resist them, they should be carefully considered before sending the paper elsewhere. A paper rejected twice should be examined particularly carefully; it is probably scientifically weak or poorly presented or both. Rather than try a third journal think about preparing a shortened version or making a contribution to a related debate through a correspondence column.

The current emphasis on more concise scientific papers has created difficulties in selecting how much detail to give or omit regarding methods, results and discussion. The priorities will vary from topic to topic and journal to journal and this is a further reason for studying the house-style of the journal of your choice, as well as for asking colleagues' views on whether your mix of detail is the right one. A final point relates to the submission of a rejected paper to a second journal. Have it retyped; nothing is so obvious as a paper which has previously been on two postal journeys and read by several scrutineers.

Contributions to correspondence are normally shorter than formal articles but, as they do not require summaries or introductions, still leave considerable scope for presenting material which may not be of sufficient quantity or quality to merit an independent paper.

In all writing it is wise to observe the courtesies expected of a professional. No matter how outraged you may be by a point of view it is surely possible to start a reply be referring for example to 'Dr X's interesting and provocative article' in preference to indulging in invective or sarcasm, both of which lower the standing of the attacker and stimulate sympathy for the attacked. In the same way a dignified silence in response to personalised attack may be remembered longer than even a well-reasoned reply.

When you have had an article accepted – and most editors will welcome any well-written and carefully reasoned presentation from general practice – you will still have one duty left, namely proof reading. This should be done thoroughly as careless mistakes in an article detract from its effect, particularly when they involve numerical errors (for example, tables which don't add up properly), inconsistencies between tables and text, incorrect references, absent negatives and sentences which don't convey sense because of a missing verb. These errors are only too easily missed when reading a familiar text.

Writing a Thesis

A thesis for a higher degree normally reflects a substantial involvement in a research field over a number of years. The decision to embark on a thesis is usually taken after an initial research project has been completed and has stimulated a wish to probe more widely or more deeply into the field of interest. The time taken over research leading to a thesis varies from as little as one or two years to ten or more. My own view is that about four years is desirable and at the same time long enough to spend on any one interest before changing to a new topic or substantially different aspect of the original topic; the writer of a thesis should aim to complete his work within five years if at all possible. But even a much shorter time spent on the wrong lines can of course become wasted time and may lead to submission of a thesis which fails because of scientific inadequacy. In recent years the submission of an increasing number of scientifically weak theses has caused many universities to insist that prospective candidates register their field of interest, and in some cases identify named supervisors acceptable to the university. When a doctor sees a research interest developing well he should ask himself whether he is interested in and willing to undertake the work involved in preparing a thesis. If so, he should make preliminary enquiries of colleagues knowledgeable on the subject of writing a thesis and find out the detailed requirements of his own university. Williams (1974) has listed some of the topics which have produced MDs from general practice and Richardson (1975) has written guide notes on working for the degree. The RCGP Library has copies of many theses from general practice and universities hold copies of theses which have been awarded passes by them. It is worth looking at one or two; their diversity of topic and length is more noteworthy than any consistencies which will be found.

In contrast to a published paper where only selected references and results are normally presented, and the discussion is inevitably restricted in its depth, the thesis requires rigorous review of literature, detailed presentation and defence of experimental design and method, and a thorough discussion of the findings and their implications. A thesis containing 100 references, 100 pages (20,000-25,000 words) and perhaps 25 tables and illustrations will keep most examiners happy. There is no intrinsic merit in length!

This is not the place to argue the value of writing a thesis; but any doctor who accepts the challenge and complies in good faith with its demands will gain a new respect for the vastness of knowledge which already exists and quickly realise the smallness of the amount which any one project or any one person can add to it.

Writing is the more formal and disciplined part of the responsibility which the research worker has to communicate and publicise his findings. The next chapter aims to help the doctor who wishes or is willing to talk about his research.

References

Richardson, I.M., 'MD in General Practice – an Introduction', *Update*, 10 (1975), pp.1141-5.

Thorne, C., *Thorne's Better Medical Writing*, 2nd edn. (Pitman Medical, Tunbridge Wells, 1977).

Williams, W.O., 'MD by Thesis from General Practice', *Journal of the Royal College of General Practitioners*, 24 (1974), pp.778-83.

15 SPEAKING ABOUT RESEARCH

General practice includes in its ranks many notable raconteurs and persuasive political orators, but sadly in the decade following the 1966 Charter the dependence of general practice on the consultant postgraduate lecture prevented many family doctors from developing talents as lecturers on clinical and scientific topics. However, attitudes to postgraduate education have changed in the last few years and the general practitioner now has many more opportunities to speak about his work. Too often these openings are left unfilled or are filled unsatisfactorily. The reasons for reluctance to speak are understandable – inexperience, anxiety about telling colleagues how to do their own job, fear of a hostile reception or being unable to answer questions, awareness of incomplete knowledge of a field and the possible superior knowledge of individuals in the audience. Don't be put off; anyone with something new or interesting to say can be assured of a friendly and grateful reception from his colleagues. Remember that the lecturer's job is to stimulate interest and discussion and not to provide all the answers. As with any worthwhile skill, the ability to speak well depends on a mixture of natural aptitude, training and experience. This chapter aims to help the inexperienced speaker make the most of his natural talents. Speaking is a very individual activity and different styles are right for different people. Some of the suggestions I make in this chapter are personal ones although many apply generally. Anyone wanting to improve his ability as a speaker should watch others for good and bad features of delivery and model himself on the mix that suits his theme of interest and personality. Successful speaking gives the same enjoyment as holing a long putt to beat your local consultant surgeon on the last green; unsuccessful speaking is like taking three putts from four feet. There are ways of making the first more likely than the second!

Reading a Paper

A formal paper may be given in any of a wide range of circumstances. Contributions may last anywhere from five minutes (avoid this – it is educationally hopeless as well as a bit of an insult to both you and your audience) to fifty minutes (which is equivalent to at least two full-length church sermons!). Audiences may be lay or professional, and if professional may be drawn from widely different groups with very different experience of medicine in general and general practice in particular. Facilities for speaking may range from excellent to dreadful or inappropriate – for example, an audience of ten in a lecture room designed for 150. There may or may not be opportunities for questions, you may or may not be the only speaker and you may or may not be the person with the first or the last word.

Preparation

All satisfactory communications to any audience depend on the care given to preparation. This applies to everyone although the experienced speaker may be distinguished from the novice by his ability to prepare adequately at very short notice. Rarely is an unprepared communication any more than barely adequate; it is likely to be confusing, to run over or under time, to be inappropriately illustrated, to irritate the audience and to (rightly) damage the reputation of the speaker. 'Preparation' includes time spent over many weeks or years in thinking about a topic and how to present it, and should not be seen as restricted to the time spent writing notes for a particular talk or session. Be sceptical about the speaker who says he has not prepared his talk and proceeds to talk impressively – and certainly do not use this approach as a personal policy.

Preparation for a talk includes many things: knowing how long to speak; finding out how many are expected to be present and the nature of the audience; finding out exactly where one will be speaking and what facilities will be available; checking as to what are the aims of the meeting, course or session; finding out who else is speaking and what each has been asked to say (not always of course the same as what each is actually going to say) and enquiring what plans have been made for discussion.

Try to decide precisely what you want members of your audience to remember. Realise that they will take away only a few factual items and that they may remember more clearly a single point of philosophy or attitude. The most important educational opportunity may be the chance to show the audience, for example, the self-critical approach of the apparently easy-going rural doctor or the concern felt by a harassed city doctor over a particular aspect of the social implications of his daily work. Or it may be a demonstration of how absorbing research can be or a demonstration of the difference between association of observation and a proof of cause and effect. Decide on no more than three themes (or aims) for your talk. Plan to tell your audience what these are early in your presentation; then develop your themes according to the time available and the characteristics of your audience and finally, in good time, summarise what you have been saying and end by restating your original aims.

The choice between speaking from a script or from notes has to be made early in preparation. Where a talk involves close reasoning and precise use of words, or centres round the development of a philosophical theme, a prepared script is the only safe way of guaranteeing that you will say exactly what you want to say. Having a script available gives valuable reassurance to a speaker and, of course, does not mean that it has to be used throughout a talk. When the audience is large, the occasion formal, or the paper of precise scientific importance, the greater the need will be for the use of a script. On the other hand total dependence on a script inevitably constrains the speaker and generally reduces spontaneity; it can hinder the achievement of rapport with an audience and reduces the chances of the audience identifying with the speaker's attitudes as well as accepting his science – which may be unfortunate. Dependence on a script may produce a completely inappropriate result such as reading a talk to an audience of a dozen – the nadir of educational achievement. For the purposes of most general practice lecturing occasions, I prepare a series of headings on 8in. x 5in. postcards – printed in block capitals. This reminds me of the points I want to develop and the order and relative importance of each. Below or at the side of each heading I list three or four points I hope to make and the numbers of any slides I want to show. If the topic is one on which I have spoken before the notes will be relatively few; if the topic is a new one, they will be more extensive. Occasionally the scientific 'meat' in the middle is presented between a more philosophical introduction and conclusion and it may be appropriate to deliver the introductory part from a script. Some topics will be illustrated with slides which themselves can substitute for notes and this is a convenient technique for use as an *aide-memoire.* It is worth remembering that if slides are to be used they will probably be shown in a darkened room which may make reading even from a well-lit lectern a difficult task.

Special attention should be given to the opening part of an address and to the closing stages. It is important to make a good first impression with your audience and this is often made difficult by the inevitable nervousness which is experienced by most speakers on most occasions. Start with a few informal and personal remarks; this helps to relax both you and your audience and helps them to identify positively with you.

Write your opening sentences in full in your notes and refer to them immediately before starting to talk. Give equal thought to the finish and again write your final passage on your note cards or script to guarantee the right ending.

Even if I am talking on a subject on which I have spoken regularly I always rewrite my notes for each individual talk. And no matter how well I think I know any topic and how totally I may appear to be independent of notes, they are always somewhere accessible if required. Once again do not believe those who claim not to prepare. . .and do not attempt to imitate. Remember that the best extempore speeches are normally the best prepared!

When timing has to be precise a rehearsal may help; a talk given live is usually given quicker than in rehearsal. An A4 page of script contains around 250 words and a delivery rate of 120 words per minute is about average. Allow between one and two minutes for each slide to be shown. Make sure that any script is readable; avoid having to change pages in mid-sentence. Asterisk key starting points if you may be moving to and from your script and do not prepare a script in a crowded manner or on both sides of a page.

Giving the Talk

Turn up on good time, looking tidy and apparently looking forward to the occasion. . .and stone-cold sober! Try to meet your chairman and fellow speakers and perhaps one or two of the audience to gauge the 'feel' of the occasion. Ask who will be and who will not be present with a view to avoiding unfortunate throw-away remarks which although harmless nine times out of ten are out of place the tenth time – like illustrating a point by reference to an unfortunate characteristic which happens to be possessed by the person who is to propose the vote of thanks! Find out who may ask awkward questions and who is the local expert on your topic. Ask about acoustics; try out lights and switches; find out if the microphone works; meet the projectionist and get clear the projection arrangements for the session; load your own slides if possible – checking the order of your slides (again!) and see that the projection is in focus. Walk round the hall to assess the viewing angles – where can you stand without impeding the view of your screen. If you are not due to speak until late in a programme sit near the back. You will be able to absorb the atmosphere of the meeting best from there – and escape to relieve yourself if the need should arise.

When the moment to speak arrives approach the lectern slowly and steady yourself before starting. Make sure the audience has had a brief break between speakers and that everyone has settled again before you start. Look at the audience; appear to recognise that they exist; smile, greet them and acknowledge the chairman. This gives you a start and establishes communication; it also helps to identify and speak to someone towards the back of the audience; if you can see that people near the back are listening the audience is probably still with you. Make your opening remarks positive and avoid at all costs saying you don't know why you have been asked or that you have nothing particularly interesting to say, or that you thought about your talk last night for the first time. If you make such remarks your audience and hosts will be entitled to feel fools for asking you, or for coming to listen to you. A little pleasant humour is always an asset, but avoid funny stories (unless really apt) and in particular avoid blue stories, religious stories and other themes liable to cause offence.

Irrespective of the length of your talk, tell your audience what you hope to achieve early in your address and remember that few new ideas will be absorbed after the first ten minutes. Where an address is to last longer than twenty minutes break it into sections separating each for example, by some clinical illustrations or by showing a few slides, or by a bit of informal chat, or by a change of position at the lectern. Although I have suggested fixing on a member of the audience, do not stick with one person throughout; remember that there are two sides to a room and a back and a front. If you feel that the audience is being lost – two people talking or someone clearly bored or asleep – speak to or at the individual concerned for the next few sentences, raising your voice a bit, speaking a bit faster or moving physically closer to the audience. Remember it is easier to keep hold of an audience than to regain attention once lost. Audiences are readily bored by too many tables, too much theory, too many statistics or too many points of detail. Attention is also difficult to hold immediately before lunch, at the end of the day, and late in the evening. Audiences sedated by over-generous hospitality, although seeming initially receptive, are often hard to keep interested; they also tend to be less constructive in their criticism afterwards.

Other suggestions are common sense: do not turn your back on the audience; do not mumble into notes; do not rattle money and keys in your pocket or charge around the room like a clockwork soldier. Avoid repetitive gestures with the hands and the use of recurrent phrases, all of which distract attention. In this respect nothing is more valuable than advice from a friend or colleague – these habits develop unconsciously and soon become difficult to shake off if not corrected.

Finally, avoid running over time; to do so reduces the opportunities for the questions and discussion which a good talk should generate, and holds up arrangements for later speakers, meals and so on. In certain settings speakers who run over time may be asked to close without completing their papers – an experience reputed to be acutely embarrassing! Apart from being poor technique, too long a paper rarely interests as much as one of the length requested or one a little shorter than expected.

Question Time

Many speakers are apprehensive about questions after a paper, but when a speaker is presenting his own work and is prepared to admit or concede doubtful ground to reasoned argument, he should have nothing to worry about. It is unwise to attempt to answer questions you have not understood and equally unwise to 'flannel' when a weakness or error in your material is identified. Willingness to give straightforward YES or NO answers is always appreciated by audiences and the effect of a paper is enhanced by apparent openness in its discussion. Whether as a speaker or as a questioner it is proper to be critical of methods, results, or interpretation of research, but unwise to criticise colleagues at a personal level. Audiences will quickly rally to support someone under personal attack from either side of the rostrum. Dignified silence under such pressure is a strong weapon; avoid angling to achieve the 'last word' which is often trivial and thus counter-productive. Some speakers use the technique of reflecting questions back to the questioner, but this also is liable to misfire when arguing with a capable adversary. Take time to consider answers to difficult questions, and try to keep the initiative – perhaps by standing and moving forwards to answer a difficult question or to make an important point. Whether as questioner or responder, avoid giving a lecture in preface or in reply to a question.

Visual Aids

Most scientific papers are improved when good illustrations are used properly. Slides (2in. x 2in. mounted transparencies) remain the commonest visual aid in use, although the overhead projector (or OHP) is proving a popular alternative because of the ease with which speakers can prepare their own material.

Evans (1978) has summarised the qualities of good visual material as 'appropriate, accurate, legible, comprehensible, well-executed, interesting and memorable'. Just as well-prepared material enhances a communication so does bad material reduce its impact. Many doctors practise within range of a hospital which will help with production of visual material and can choose between slides and overhead projection. For doctors with limited or no access to help, overhead projection will usually be the best solution. Many of the common faults of visual material reflect lack of guidance in preparation and differentiate the amateur from the professional approach to public speaking. (Some believe that the amateur approach is more homely and that to be 'professional' has an off-putting effect on general practitioners; I can only disagree.) The following suggestions may help when deciding what visual material to prepare or use.

1. Illustrations aim to focus attention and emphasise points; ten slides are probably as many as should be used in any one talk. Where serial pictures are used to build an argument, a summary slide can concentrate the impact. Just as it is helpful to list conclusions at the start as well as at the finish of a paper, the use of a summary slide at start and finish is often useful.
2. Too many slides include too much material. Four columns and three rows of figures is as much as can be taken in at a time and accompanying script reduces impact. General practice audiences tend to be less numerate than those who speak to them and figures may have less impact than the lecturer hopes. Avoid redundant material like details of statistical tests and percentages with decimal places; add necessary detail orally when the slide is shown. Eight lines of information has been suggested as a limit when script is being used.
3. Give your audience time to look at each slide before you talk about it; and leave it on for a few seconds afterwards for the message to be appreciated and for notes to be taken if wished. Address the audience and not the slide; when using a pointer place the end firmly on the screen to avoid casting a shadow or double image; 'torch' pointers are often difficult to see and exaggerate any nervous tremors! They also distract an audience if the arrow is allowed to dart all over the wall and ceiling of the lecture theatre as the speaker talks.
4. I like my slides to seem specific to the talk I am giving. I thus avoid heading slides as *slide 1, slide 2* and so on; not only is useful space on the slide wasted but the scope of the slide is compromised. A talk which starts with *slide 9* and then shows Table XIV and then *slide 3* creates an impression of being impersonal and mass-produced.

5. When preparing material for slides or the OHP use all space available. Unlike journal productions, space at the margins and edges is wasted. Ordinary typewriters do not always prepare good slides; special type is available for preparation of material for projection and 'lettraset' transfers help in making OHP transparencies (otherwise normally prepared by felt-pen on commercially available acetate paper). Slides fade with time, burn out in the centre with overuse and, like OHP material, become dirty. This also creates an undistinguished effect and such material should be renewed.
6. Print rather than write on OHP plates. Sheets of acetate paper can be mounted in frames. This prevents preparations curling due to heat from the projector: curling leads to gradual production of a double or triple image at the edges during projection. Remember that unless an overhead projector projects on to a matching angled screen, distortion of the image will occur.
7. Few people can write on an OHP and speak at the same time. The effect of trying both is usually verbally and/or visually untidy!
8. Some speakers use 'impact' slides for the purpose implied. These include cartoons, holiday pictures, and a variety of unexpected flashes of widely ranging relevance. When this is well done (tastefully and in good proportion and usually by a genuinely skilled speaker) the effect can be excellent. Badly used, they are distracting and often draw attention to fundamental weaknesses in the basic presentation; probably the technique is best restricted to use of a single opening or concluding slide.
9. A speaker whose talk depends on his slides or other illustrative material should have contingency plans available for the event of machine failure. Many speakers carry a spare projector bulb – others a spare talk!
10. Read Evans, *British Medical Journal*, 1 (1978), p.905!

I would like to close with a word on behalf of a dying but valuable old friend – the blackboard and chalk. No better aid for building a lecture has been found and its skilful use is much to be recommended particularly for small group teaching. It should only be used to build a visual and semi-permanent summary and its unplanned use can be as unsatisfactory as misuse of the other techniques already described. Handout summary sheets should be considered as a supplement to the use of either the blackboard or any of the other methods described above. These are particularly likely to be useful when lectures are aimed at educational rather than research purposes.

Reference

Evans, M., 'The Abuse of Slides', *British Medical Journal*, 1 (1978), pp.905-8.

16 POSTSCRIPT

The four parts of this book have presented the development of research from its beginnings as an unanswered question to its conclusion as a well-constructed reasoned scientific paper. In the first part, I have suggested that an interest be allowed to develop gradually through the stages from asking a question to posing a hypothesis or listing aims for study. During this time there is literature to be read, advice and the opinions of others to be sought, and the need to live with the idea for long enough to be sure that it is of real interest. The second part of the sequence involves planning the study. Attention has to be given to the quality of information which will be required and seems likely to be available, and to the quantity of information needed and how it is to be found. Financial implications, requirements for specialist assistance from the laboratory, the statistician and the data processor and ethical implications, all need to be thought through, and the choice of whether to involve other colleagues has to be made. After the fieldwork is complete, information must be classified and coded, 'processed' by hand or machine, tabulated and interpreted. Finally, comes the task of preparing a report for publication and perhaps presenting the findings to one's colleagues locally, or further afield. The three chapters which I have included to show how the principles of research are modified and applied in practice also try to show that research is capable of creating the same emotions and feelings of involvement as is experienced in many other forms of clinical work. In this concluding chapter, I want to draw attention to some problems which I believe have to be faced before general practice research can make its full contribution to helping the development of the health and social services in this country.

General Practice and Research

Research has for long been a valued activity in the established disciplines of hospital medicine. Indeed, the current pattern has been for new disciplines to evolve in response to advances in knowledge made possible by new research findings in a parent discipline. Bacteriology, for example, developed from pathology and now virology has developed from bacteriology; in the same way gastroenterology and nephrology are two of many special fields which have evolved from general medicine, and neurosurgery and orthopaedic surgery are sub-specialties of general surgery. Research developments in new specialties often precede the provision of new clinical services, which in turn create opportunities and needs for teaching, first in the postgraduate field and later to undergraduates.

The basic science research component of the discipline (now often described as 'biomedical' research) then continues to be developed by those with particular abilities in the more scientific aspects of research and increasingly this involves skill in the fields of, for example, biochemistry, immunology and genetics. The applied science research component ('health services research') is developed by those whose major involvement in the discipline is a clinical one, or by those with skill in epidemiological research. The applied science attempts to interpret the basic science in terms of the needs of the community at large. From combining the results of applied and basic science research it should be possible to comment on important issues including needs of communities, allocation of resources and quality of care. But for the information on these issues to be of value the 'basic science' available must be both correct and complete.

It is difficult to apply this model to general practice, but helpful to try. The clinical boundaries of general practice have been determined by a complex mixture of historical, political and social factors, rather than in response to developments in any one field of physiological or pathological research. Now its attempts to map out and define its role are being complicated by the need to use one set of measuring techniques and values (those of the clinical scientist) at its border with hospital medicine, and a different set of techniques and values (those of the social scientist) when studying the boundary between non-professional self-care and professional primary care. Neither general practice nor general practice research has yet come to terms with the need to compromise between the more numerical and quantitative requirements of clinical research and clinical decision making (the 'science') and the less numerate and more qualitative emphases of the behavioural or social scientist (the 'art'). It is thus premature to see general practice research as being able to contribute effectively to determining priorities and standards of care within the health and social services generally, although this must eventually be the contribution which general practice research is uniquely placed to offer.

If we return to the traditional model of the evolution of a discipline, we must surely face the truth that many of the difficulties we presently encounter in attempting to do applied research in general practice and to define 'quality of care' stem from the absence of sufficient understanding of the 'basic science' of our discipline.

I have earlier suggested that three triangles summarised the more important relationships which had to be evaluated before the 'basic science' of general practice could be regarded as adequately understood.

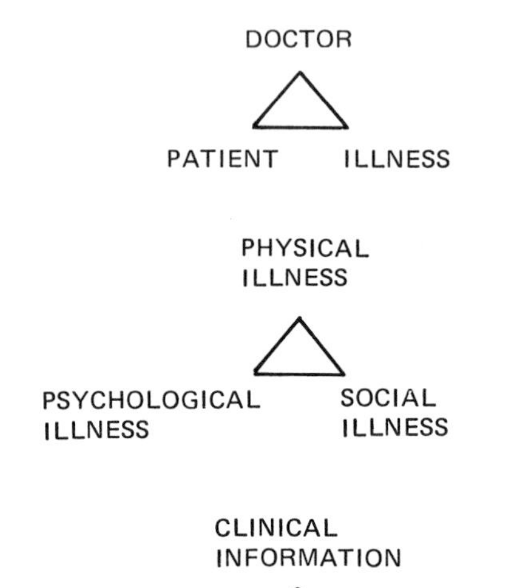

Until these relationships have been studied to a greater depth than is the case at present it will not be possible to acknowledge quantitatively the wide range of ways in which the 'art' and the 'science' may be combined to provide good general practice service care; in consequence the basis for clinical care, teaching and future research will remain disquietingly subjective. The logical conclusion to the emphasis I have placed on the need for careful study of the deeper implications of what happens at individual consultations, is that I want to support and encourage thoughtful and careful research by individual general practitioners working with their own patients, in their own practices. Although large-scale, multi-doctor studies have important contributions to make to many aspects of research in general practice, they cannot, I believe, provide the basis for this type of fundamentally important research.

The key question to be faced by those now deciding the direction of general practice research – in universities, in the RCGP, in the health departments – is how best to balance their support of these complementary styles of research. In the 'sixties' the multi-observer type of study was particularly helpful, while the nature of the work of general practice was being outlined for the first time; in the 'eighties' the emphasis must, I think, shift to encourage more detailed and perceptive analyses of the consultation between the doctor and his patient.

The General Practitioner and Research

By tradition, general practice is seen as a job to be 'got on with' rather than thought about in numerical terms and this philosophy has saved the health service from much embarrassment in the past. It is also a tradition with its limitations and these limitations are exposed when teaching is required or standards of care are being discussed. These pressures are now with the general practitioner – from trainees and students on the one hand, and his patients and the public on the other – and they are not likely to go away conveniently.

I would like to introduce one final triangle of activities and suggest

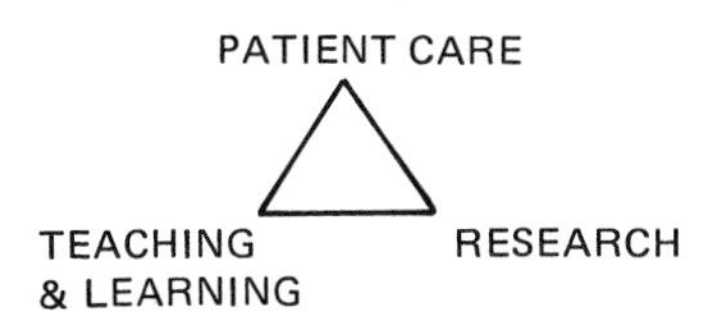

that these activities of service work, education and research are as closely interdependent as are the other aspects of general practice care I have linked together earlier in this chapter. The hypotheses on which I have based this monograph are:

> that the prospering of general practice as an independent discipline depends on a wider recognition of the importance of this relationship; and
> that the individual doctor consciously or unconsciously depends on the integrity of this triangle for the continued development of his daily work.

No one would suggest that it is necessary to do research, either to teach or to practice. It is, however, important that the practitioner or teacher keeps effective contacts with opportunities to hear about and discuss research work which might affect his daily work. Even if the doctor is not personally involved in research at first hand, participation in the discipline of research thinking remains the most valuable and practical way of ensuring that clinical observations, assessments and actions will be kept keen, perceptive and appropriate. And it is this that makes doctors ask the kind of questions about their daily work which starts off the research process which this book describes.

APPENDIX

Selected Reading

Some facts and figures about general practice
Trends in General Practice 1977 (Royal College of General Practitioners, London, 1977)

A different way of thinking about familiar problems
de Bono, E., *The Use of Lateral Thinking* (Cape, London, 1976)

Some commonly used research terms
'A general practice glossary', *Journal of the Royal College of General Practitioners*, supplement 3 to vol.23 (1973)

A guide to the preparation of questionnaires
Bennett, A.E. & Ritchie, K., *Questionnaires in Medicine* (Oxford University Press, London, 1975)

Methods of compiling disease indexes
Eimeral, T.S. & Laidlaw, A.J., *A Handbook for Research in General Practice* (E. & S. Livingstone, London & Edinburgh, 1969)

Advice on where to seek funding for research
Research Funds Guide, 3rd edn. (British Medical Association, London, 1976)

A simple guide to the principles of medical statistics
Swinscow, T.D.V., *Statistics at Square One* (British Medical Journal, London, 1976)

A more detailed discussion of statistical method
Hill, A.B., *Principles of Medical Statistics*, 9th edn. (The Lancet, London, 1971)

A guide to the principles of medical writing and speaking
Thorne's Better Medical Writing, 2nd edn. (Pitman Medical, Tunbridge Wells, 1977)

The Six Projects

Project 1: 'Early or Late Antibiotics in a Flu Epidemic?' (pp.50, 101, 155)

The clinical trial was reported under the title:

'Double-blind trial of early demethylchlortetracycline in minor respiratory illness in general practice', Howie, J.G.R. & Clark, G.A., *Lancet*, 2 (1970), pp.1099-102.

Project 2: 'Do "Diagnoses" Determine or Justify Management Decisions?' (pp.52, 108, 157)

Two papers were published using information from this study:

'Diagnosis – the Achilles heel', *Journal of the Royal College of General Practitioners*, 22 (1972), pp.310-15. 'A new look at respiratory illness in general practice', *Journal of the Royal College of General Practitioners*, 23 (1973), pp.895-904.

Project 3: 'Co-trimoxazole and Streptococcal Tonsillitis' (pp.54, 112, 159)

A contribution based on this work appeared in the correspondence columns of the *British Medical Journal*:

'Drug monitoring and adverse reactions', *British Medical Journal*, 1 (1977), p.1467.

Project 4: 'The Prevention of Adverse Drug Reactions' (pp.55, 115, 160)

The evaluation of the drug-interaction warning labels was reported as shown:

'Prevention of adverse drug interactions', Howie, J.G.R., Jeffers, T.A., Millar, H.R. & Petrie, J.C., *British Journal of Clinical Pharmacology*, 4 (1977), pp.611-14.

Project 5: 'Can Clinical Judgement Be Analysed?' (pp.58, 117, 161)

The project designed to examine this question was described under the heading:

'Clinical judgement and antibiotic use in general practice', *British Medical Journal*, 2 (1976), pp.1061-4.

Project 6: 'Prescribing to Save Work' (pp.60, 124, 163)

The results of this retrospective study of practice records were presented in a 'short report':

'Antibiotics and respiratory illness in general practice: prescribing policy and work load', Howie, J.G.R. & Hutchison, K.R., *British Medical Journal*, 2 (1978), p.1342.

General Assistance

Help with references and reviewing literature

The Librarian, The Royal College of General Practitioners, 14 Princes Gate, London SW7 1PU.

Cards for an age-sex register

Birmingham Research Unit (RCGP), Lordswood House, 54 Lordswood Road, Harborne, Birmingham 17.

Advice on research either in general terms or in relation to individual projects can be obtained through the RCGP, whose range of services is listed in its Annual Report, *or* through any university department of general practice.

INDEX

Footnote: practical examples are included in appropriate chapters and in the illustrative material in Chapters 6, 10, 13 (see pp.190-1).